Homeopathic
First Aid
for Animals

Homeopathic First Aid for Animals

TALES AND TECHNIQUES FROM A COUNTRY PRACTITIONER

KAETHERYN WALKER

Illustrated by Cheryl Adam

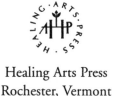

Healing Arts Press
Rochester, Vermont

Healing Arts Press
One Park Street
Rochester, Vermont 05767
www.gotoit.com

Note to the reader: This book is intended as an informational guide. The remedies, approaches, and techniques described herein are meant to supplement, and not to be a substitute for, professional veterinary care or treatment. They should not be used to treat a serious ailment without prior consultation with a state-licensed veterinarian.

LIBRARY OF CONGRESS CATALOGING-IN-PUBLICATION DATA
Walker, Kaetheryn. 1956–
    Homeopathic first aid for animals : tales and techniques from a country practitioner / Kaetheryn
       Walker.
     p. cm.
    Includes bibliographical references and index.
    ISBN 0-89281-737-2 (alk. paper)
    1. Homeopathic veterinary medicine—Handbooks, manuals, etc. 2. First aid for animals—
       Handbooks, manuals, etc. I. Title.
    SF746.W35 1997
    636.089'5532—dc21   97-18370
                                                  CIP

Printed and bound in Canada
10 9 8 7 6 5 4 3 2 1

Text design and layout by Virginia L. Scott
This book was typeset in Garamond with Wiesbaden Swing and Lithos as the display typefaces

Healing Arts Press is a division of Inner Traditions International

Distributed to the book trade in Canada by Publishers Group West (PGW), Toronto, Ontario

Distributed to the health food trade in Canada by Alive Books, Toronto and Vancouver

Distributed to the book trade in the United Kingdom by Deep Books, London

Distributed to the book trade in Australia by Millennium Books, Newtown, N.S.W.

Distributed to the book trade in New Zealand by Tandem Press, Auckland

Distributed to the book trade in South Africa by Alternative Books, Ferndale

*This book is dedicated
with deep gratitude and respect to
Stephen Tobin, Dr. Med. Vet., teacher, mentor,
and dear friend, who helped me understand
that the right question is the answer.*

Contents

Preface

For many of us who share our lives with animal companions, their traumas, accidents, and illnesses are no less upsetting and dramatic than our own. The signs and symptoms of an animal in distress are very much the same as those for humans in distress: crying out, difficulty breathing or moving any body part, stupor, dizziness, vomiting, diarrhea, discharges or bleeding from a body opening or part, fever, excessive coldness of a body part, undue anxiety or fear, loss of consciousness, and unusual symptoms—both mental and physical—that come on suddenly. Any of these symptoms may be caused by accidents that you may witness. Less noticeable causes may include events you may not witness firsthand, such as poisonings, insect bites, punctures, or territory disputes with other animals, to name a few.

But as dramatic as all this sounds, you can make a big difference in the well-being of your animal companion. With the proper information and tools at your disposal, you will be able to handle almost any emergency situation involving your animal companion. Being well prepared, informed, and calm will give you an edge that may well save your animal companion's life in the event of a serious emergency.

As with any illness or accident requiring first aid, it is in everyone's best interest for you to be familiar with what to do and how to do it. For this reason it is recommended that you read through this manual before an emergency situation arises. Familiarize yourself with the layout of the manual, the names of the remedies, the first-aid techniques, and the symptoms unique to each remedy.

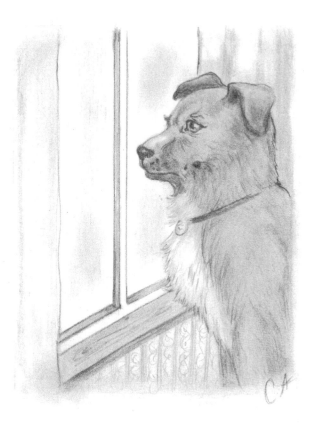

It is also important to jot down, inside the front cover of this book, the phone number of your animal's veterinarian so that it will be readily available to you in the event of an emergency. Call your veterinarian and ask if he or she is available for emergencies, which may occur during the night or on weekends or holidays. If your veterinary clinic cannot accommodate non-business-hour emergency visits, ask for a referral; if such a referral is not available from your vet, find an emergency-hours vet in your area. Find out how your emergency call will be handled. Will a recorded message be forwarded to a pager or an answering service? Will your call be immediately returned, or will there be a short waiting period? Will a vet be willing to make an emergency house call? Again, it is a good investment to be fully prepared ahead of time; you may not have the luxury of wasting precious minutes tracking down help, and the better prepared you are to handle emergencies, the better your chances of a successful outcome.

In cases of accidental poisoning of animals, advance preparation may save a life. Do take a moment to locate in chapter 29 (p. 150) the phone number for Animal Poison Control in Georgia, decide ahead of time which of the two offered phone numbers you will call if you ever need to do so, and post copies of the emergency phone numbers for both your vet and Animal Poison Control by the telephone. You may not have precious minutes to waste in this type of first aid situation.

In addition to first-aid techniques and homeopathic and supplementary care for animals, there are other important topics covered in this manual. Instructions for how to make a simple electrolyte solution are offered, as well as substitute infant milk formulas for kittens and puppies. There is also important information about how much and how frequently to feed an orphaned infant.

Homeopathic remedies can be safely and effectively used for all species of animals. Homeopathy is even applicable to birds and reptiles, and special notes on these species are included at the end of the manual.

Acknowledgments

Special thanks are due to all the animals with whom I have been blessed to work over the years. Their gentle acceptance of my desire to help, coupled with their willingness to communicate helpful messages, has taught me valuable lessons in my evolution as one who wishes to alleviate suffering.

Thanks and gratitude for all manner of help and encouragement go to Nancy Bouffard, Karen and Bill Collins, the Corbin family, Dr. Rhonda Feiman, Dianna Gould, Petra Hall, Betty Hawkins, Kathleen Kravik, Forrest Lancaster, Dianne Lee, Sand Leiser, Jeanette Maher, Pam Massey, Suzanne Richman and Goddard College, Katharine Scherer, and Martin Steingesser. I also thank Nancy Backman, who brought homeopathy to my attention at a time in my life when I despaired of finding an approach that facilitated true healing; you are present daily in my work and in my heart.

My heartfelt thanks to my agents, Cheryl Seal and David Adam, whose enthusiasm, professionalism, and conscientious responsibility brought this work to the public arena and who understood that some things are simply meant to be. Because of Cheryl's astute and intuitive insight, this book took shape in this form. Behind the scenes, and attending to every minute detail and scattered thread, David's devotion to the endless minutiae of the literary industry made this book a reality. I could not have done it without them.

Deep appreciation and gratitude go to all the folks at Inner Traditions International who made this book happen in the best way possible, especially Jon Graham, Rowan Jacobsen, Deborah Kimbell, and Christine Sumner.

Introduction

This homeopathic first-aid manual for animals was laid out for ease of use by the general public. It is not necessary to have a medical or an emergency medical technician's certificate to use it successfully. The first chapter provides guidance for treating your animal homeopathically, and chapter 2 discusses companion animal safety. Beginning with chapter 3, each chapter covers one medical topic, in alphabetical order by the name of the topic. The text of each topic chapter follows a logical sequence: it begins with an introductory statement about that particular subject, followed (where applicable) by a scenario involving an animal in distress. First-aid instructions are then presented, and the chapter ends with a descriptive list of symptoms and the corresponding homeopathic remedy.

At the end of chapter 1 (pp. 7 and 8) you will find a list of the thirty-two remedies referred to in this manual. The list also includes a Bach flower tincture commonly called Nature's Rescue (this product was formerly called Rescue Remedy and is also known by other names, such as Calming Essence) and the Bach Calendula tincture. This group of remedies and the one flower essence was chosen because they address a wide variety of common symptoms. Most of them can be purchased in health food stores and retail stores that focus on natural products.

All remedies are available in a variety of potencies, or strengths, the most common being 30c. The numeral 30 refers to the number of times the remedy has been diluted. The letter c indicates the ratio of the dilution of medicinal substance to dilution material, specifically, one part medicinal substance to ninety-nine parts of dilution material. Remedies are also available in "x" potencies, which is a lesser dilution: one part medicinal substance to nine parts of dilution material. Remedies of c potency are more dilute than x potency remedies and are stronger in their action. It is also true that the higher the number, the more times a remedy has been diluted, and this, too, indicates stronger action. In all cases, the more dilute a remedy, the stronger its effect upon the body. In the practice of homeopathy, less is more.

The suggested list of homeopathic remedies incorporates a 30c potency, although if you choose to assemble your own remedy kit for animal use, any potency will do. It is recommended that all the remedies in a kit be of the same potency (i.e., all 6x or all 12c). If one has figured out the correct remedy to use in a situation, any potency will cause a curative response. Usually, low potencies (3x to 30c) act more quickly on the physical body, that is, on the cells, tissues, and organs. Higher potencies, such as 200c to 1M (M potencies are those made of 1 part medicinal substance and 999 parts dilution material), act on the emotional or mental symptoms of disease (expressed as feelings, such as apathy, sadness, or anger). Potencies above 1M affect the psychic level of disease, expressed through general psychological state, such as through phobias, fears, emotional reactivity, and mental interpretation of surroundings. These potencies are not commonly available to the general public, and their use is wisely left to the judicious prescription of a qualified homeopathic practitioner.

It is common to ask, "How do homeopathic remedies work?" Homeopathy is based on the Law of Similars, which states that "like cures like" *(similia similibus curantur)*. Simply put, a substance that causes symptoms when given in a large amount to a healthy individual will also cure similar symptoms when given in minute amounts to an ill individual. Another way to explain how homeopathic remedies work is to say that they stimulate the natural immune system to mount a defense, which results in a momentum building toward the health of the organism.

Chapter 1 discusses companion animal safety, reminding us that the ways in which we provide for our family's safety can include our animal companions. Common sense can prevent many mishaps and accidents in the first place, and the numbered list of safety suggestions is offered as a guide only. You may wish to add other safety suggestions particular to your lifestyle.

Twenty of the thirty-six topic chapters also feature short stories exemplifying a first-aid situation involving an animal. Each is intended to describe how the situation developed, what symptoms the animal had, how and why the correct remedy was chosen, and how the animal responded to that remedy. Some of the vignettes characterize situations in which qualified veterinary treatment needed to be undertaken as a follow-up. These stories are representative composites of cases I have treated in my practice as an animal homeopath over the past six years, and they represent a wide variety of animal species with which I have been privileged to work. Although the remedy(s) used in each of these vignettes is the most commonly used homeopathic remedy for the condition, each first-aid situation that you encounter will require you to *select a remedy based upon the symptoms unique to the animal.*

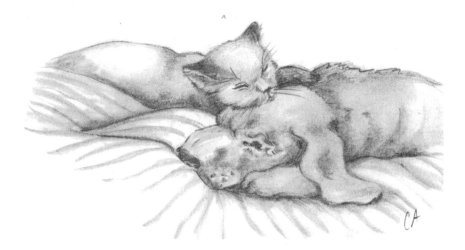

Next comes standard first-aid techniques. First aid is the aid or help initially given to an accident or illness victim until emergency medical treatment can be obtained from a qualified veterinarian. It is not, and is not intended to be, a substitute for medical care. Under no circumstances should you use this manual to diagnose or treat your animal companion's condition; only your veterinarian is qualified to do so. If you are in doubt about whether a true emergency situation exists, call a veterinarian immediately; it is far better to err on the side of caution than to risk the life of your precious animal companion.

While many first-aid techniques are listed in this manual, such as first-aid treatment for burns, electrocution, seizures, and eye injuries, this manual does not offer first-aid treatment for heart or respiratory resuscitation. The reason is that more harm can be done when attempting these procedures if you are not fully trained to perform them. Unless you have had instruction in the methods of respiratory or cardiac resuscitation, do not attempt them.

Moreover, the first-aid techniques are given in the order in which they are intended to be performed. All techniques are outlined; follow them step by step. You will not have to turn to another section to get information; any instructions you will need for a particular emergency situation are given at the beginning of each section.

Following the first-aid instructions for each topic are instructions for critical, acute, and chronic homeopathic treatment for that particular situation.

Critical situations are always life-threatening, and loss of recuperative power has already taken place; any first-aid or homeopathic remedy given should be administered on the way to a veterinary clinic, and one should seek veterinary medical help with all possible haste. Acute situations may or may not be life-threatening, but they develop with sudden and dramatic symptoms; follow-up veterinary care is strongly encouraged for all acute situations involving an animal's health. Chronic conditions show symptoms that have been around for a while; rarely are they life-threatening, and they are usually responsive to homeopathic remedies coupled with good nursing care.

A standard number of tablets or pillules to give is four. This amount varies when using very tiny granules, of which ten are equivalent to a single dose. These amounts may be given to very small animals up to animals equivalent in size to an adult human. It is recommended in the case of larger animals, such as horses, cows, or very large breeds of dogs, that one double the standard amount of tablets or pillules, in order to ensure that a full dose is given.

Following the dosage information for critical, acute, and chronic situations (and suggestions for follow-up veterinary care) are descriptions of symptoms with the corresponding homeopathic remedy. To use this section of each topic chapter, read through the symptom descriptions and choose the description that best matches the condition of the animal you are trying to help. Try to pick the remedy with symptoms most closely matching the animal's, but don't worry if it is not an exact match. Then give the corresponding remedy according to the frequency described in the instructions for critical, acute, and chronic assessment. If, after several doses, there is no response, try another remedy, the next one that most closely matches the animal's symptoms.

Use this manual in the following way:

1. Open the manual to the appropriate section.
2. Follow first-aid technique instructions in the order given. Adhere to them exactly and do not skip any procedure.
3. After using first-aid techniques, continue reading the section and follow the instructions for critical, acute, or chronic status of the situation. These descriptions will tell you whether or not you should seek medical intervention immediately or, in the case of acute or chronic situations, how frequently to give a dose of one of the remedies listed at the end of the section. Follow instructions for critical, acute, or chronic conditions to the letter; do not skip any instructions. If you are told to *seek veterinary attention immediately*, do so. Or you may be told to consult your vet only in the event your animal does not respond to your homeopathic remedy or supplement.
4. After assessing the animal's status (critical, acute, or chronic), skim through the symptoms for each remedy listed and choose the remedy that matches the animal's symptoms. Give doses according to instructions for critical, acute, or chronic and follow with any supplementary treatments, if suggested.

CHAPTER 1

How to Give Remedies to Animals

There are several simple ways to give remedies to your animal companion. Do not handle the remedy. Count out the correct number of tablets or pellets into the cover and then dispense them from the container cover into the animal's mouth or into a small container if dissolving in distilled water.

If an animal is conscious and not too upset, place the appropriate number of pellets or tablets in the cheek pouch and allow them to dissolve. Pellets or tablets may be given whole or crushed in a fold of clean white paper and the powder poured into the cheek pouch or on the tongue.

Some animals may vigorously resist being medicated. Remedies are made in a base of milk sugar and easily dissolve in milk; if an animal likes milk, this may be an alternative way of giving remedies. Another trick, especially helpful with animals who are extremely agitated, is to dip your fingers into the water dilution and flick the droplets into the animal's face (you can apologize later!). Remedies are readily absorbed by any mucous membrane, and contact with eyes, nose, or mouth will have an effect. One can easily dispense a drop or two directly into an animal's eye (at least once and if you're quick), and calm should be somewhat restored after the remedy has begun to work, which will facilitate administration of a second dose, if required. A drop in the eye is my preferred method of giving remedies to birds and reptiles. In any case, do not attempt to violate the animal's rights by forcing him or her to take a remedy. It is far better to wait until calm is partly restored than to give a remedy to an animal who is violently opposed to being helped. The priority is the animal's well-being, and risking further injury to the animal or the handler will only make things worse.

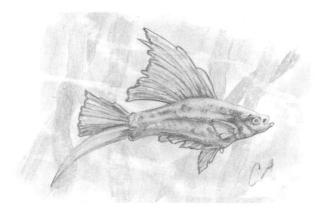

If an animal is unconscious, do not put anything in his or her mouth. Instead, dispense pellets into a clean container, add a small amount of water (about one teaspoon), and shake or stir until dissolved. Distilled water is best, but if it is unavailable, use the cleanest water you can. Then, using an eyedropper, place four drops of this dilution between the bottom lip and the gums or, even better, in the corner of the eye. Please use only plastic eyedroppers with animals; glass eyedroppers can break, or the animal may attempt to bite them. The safety and well-being of your companion animal must be a priority at all times.

REMEDIES REFERRED TO IN THIS MANUAL

ABBREVIATION	REMEDY (POTENCY)	COMMON NAME
Aconite	Aconitum napellus (30c)	Monkshood
Apis	Apis mellifica (30c)	The honeybee
Argent nit	Argentum nitricum (30c)	Silver nitrate
Arnica	Arnica montana (30c)	Leopard's bane
Ars	Arsenicum album (30c)	Arsenic trioxide

ABBREVIATION	REMEDY (POTENCY)	COMMON NAME
Bell	Belladonna (30c)	Deadly nightshade
Bry	Bryonia alba (30c)	Wild hops
Calc phos	Calcarea phosphorica (30c)	Phosphate of lime
Camph	Camphora (30c)	Camphor
Canth	Cantharis (30c)	Spanish fly
Carbo veg	Carbo vegetabilis (30c)	Vegetable charcoal
Cham	Chamomilla (30c)	German chamomile
Cocc	Cocculus indicus (30c)	Indian cockle seed
Coloc	Colocynth (30c)	Bitter cucumber
Gels	Gelsemium sempervirens (30c)	Yellow jasmine
Hepar sulph	Hepar sulphuris calcarea (6x)	Calcium sulphide
Hyper	Hypericum (30c)	Saint John's wort
Lach	Lachesis muta (30c)	Bushmaster
Ledum	Ledum palustre (30c)	Marsh-tea
Merc	Mercurius vivus (30c)	Quicksilver
Nat mur	Natrum muriaticum (30c)	Sodium chloride
Nux vom	Nux vomica (30c)	Poison nut
Phos	Phosphorus (30c)	Phosphorus
Pulex	Pulex irritans (30c)	Common flea
Puls	Pulsatilla nigricans (30c)	Pasque flower
Rhus tox	Rhus toxicodendron (30c)	Poison ivy
Ruta	Ruta graveolens (30c)	Rue-bitterwort
Staph	Staphysagria (30c)	Stavesacre
Sulph	Sulphur (30c)	Sulphur
Symph	Symphytum (30c)	Comfrey/knitbone
Urt urens	Urtica urens (30c)	Stinging nettle
Uva	Uva ursi (30c)	Bearberry
(Bach flower essence)	Nature's Rescue (tincture)	Combination of 1c potencies of the flower essences of *Helianthemum nummularium, Clematis vitalba, Impatiens glandulfera,* and *Ornithogal umumbellatum* in an alcohol base.
	Calendula tincture	Tincture of marigold flowers

CHAPTER 2

Accident Prevention

"Safety first" is a common slogan. It is generally attributed to human safety in the workplace, but it is valuable advice for the home and for our animal family members too. Too often we say in hindsight, "If only I had . . ." But this does not have to be the case. You can prevent many accidents involving your beloved animal companion from ever happening.

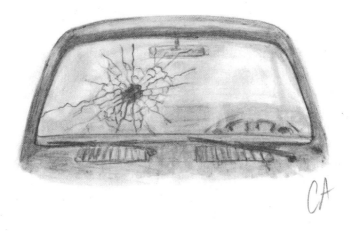

KEEPING YOUR ANIMAL COMPANION SAFE

Preventing emergency situations is the best way to keep your animal companion safe and happy. Here is a common sense list that, if incorporated into daily life with your animal companion, may prevent you from ever having to use this manual.

1. Know where your animal is at all times.
2. Keep medicines and chemicals out of reach.
3. *Never* let your animal ride in the back of an open truck. *Never!!!*
4. Put food and water bowls in safe places only; never place them near electrical cords, electrical outlets, or stoves.
5. Tack down lose rugs and carpets.
6. Don't let animals run on wet floors.
7. Keep pot handles on stoves turned inward.
8. Keep oven doors closed.
9. Check the dryer before starting (cats like to sleep there).
10. If your dog or cat is outside in summer, be sure it has shade to protect it from sunburn and plenty of fresh water. Like humans, animals can succumb to sunburn and heatstroke or dehydration.
11. Under no circumstances should you ever leave an animal in a parked car or truck in either summer or winter, even if the windows are partly or fully opened. In the summer the air inside any vehicle can heat to alarming temperatures in a matter of minutes, whether the vehicle is parked in the sun or the shade.
12. If your dog or cat is outside in the winter, make sure that it has shelter. Doghouses should be raised off the ground and supplied with hay or rugs/blankets for insulation and a covering for the door.
13. *Never* leave a cat or dog outside at night in the winter if the temperature is below thirty-two degrees Fahrenheit.
14. Practice fire drills with your family *and* include your animal companion in the drill practices. Always have two planned escape routes from anywhere in your house.
15. Keep a copy of your emergency phone number list by your phone at all times.

CHAPTER 3

Abscesses

Cats are prone to getting abscesses, usually as the result of puncture wounds from fighting or bites from other cats. Horses get abscesses, too, typically in their hooves or on their hocks, from stepping on nails or scraping against barbed wire. Dogs and rabbits get abscesses as well, but less frequently than cats or horses. Whatever the species, the experience of having an abscess can range from merely uncomfortable to downright painful. Caught early, treated with common household hydrogen peroxide, and followed up with the right homeopathic remedy, an abscess can be dealt with easily and will heal quickly.

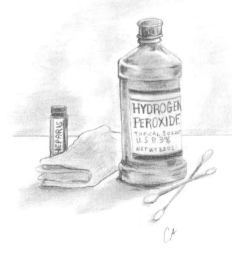

YOU'RE WELCOME!

Big Head, as we affectionately called him, was another in a long line of stray tomcats that haunted the barn behind our farmhouse. Gigantic and all muscle, he must have weighed a good twenty pounds and had a huge head, accentuated by the fact that he was a tabby cat—a breed famous for their round, bulging cheeks. We tried and tried to tame him, to bring him into the feline pride that graced our house, but to no avail.

But he would let us approach, pet him, and give him remedies when needed, and he even submitted occasionally to being picked up to be fussed over. But never for long. Within moments, he would struggle to get down, scratching and meowing, if our ministrations were too bothersome and our release not speedy enough. We were also lucky that our vet agreed to make farm calls to provide Big Head with regular immunizations, and, owing to the generous amounts of homemade cat food we gave him, he was generally healthy. Marc, the vet, had even made a house call the year before and neutered him in a makeshift surgery we'd put together in the tack room next to the horse stalls. Big Head became, in his own way, very much our cat, although it was clear that this arrangement was on his terms and his terms alone.

His greatest character defect was fighting. He determined that all of the great outdoors belonged to him, especially our property, and except for our house cats, who were puzzlingly exempt from his wrath, he would take on anything that dared trespass—big or small, fast or slow, feathered, furred, or scaled. The result was that after a night of raucous rampaging, he would disappear for a day or two, only to show up limping, usually as the result of an abscess from a bite or other puncture wound.

One early spring I found him in the loft of the barn, where he had obviously spent the night in the warmth of the hay bales. How he had climbed the ladder in the first place was a mystery, because as I watched him, he limped to the edge of the platform and looked down at me, howling. Obviously, he was in pain, and on thinking back, I reasoned that he'd climbed up there before the abscess got to the painful stage, to rest and recover. But he hadn't recovered, and now he couldn't get down.

I climbed up after him and approached cautiously. From as far away as five feet I could see the festering abscess on his left thigh; the big hole was oozing a thick, yellow-green discharge that matted below the opening. Big Head looked at me and hissed. Well, I thought, so much for the hands-on

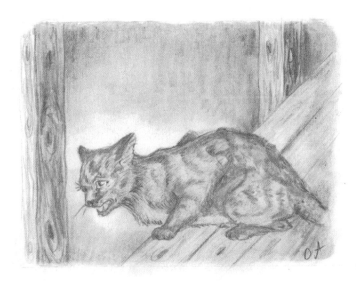

approach. In the kitchen, I mixed four pillules of Hepar sulphuris calcarea into a bowl of milk. I stirred with one hand and dialed Marc with the other.

"I can't get near him," I said in answer to Marc's query about the severity of the wound. "Of all the times he's come back with the consequences of his battles, this is by far the absolute worst. It's got to be flushed with hydrogen peroxide; maybe it'll need to be opened more, too. But unless we get him sedated, I'll never get close enough to find out. Whenever you can get here will be great. Don't forget your heavy leather gloves," I said with a chuckle. "I'll see if I can get some Nature's Rescue into him in the meantime."

Back in the barn, Big Head growled at me as I reached the top of the ladder with the Have-A-Heart trap in tow. I pushed it forward, well away from the edge of the overhang, and propped open the door. He didn't know it, but I had a plan. After the remedy began to work and he fell asleep, I planned to put him into the trap with the help of my heavy work gloves, which I had tucked into the waistband of my jeans. For now, I placed them beside a bale of hay, along with the medicated saucer of milk, and went back down to the tack room to wait.

In the stillness of the barn I heard him lapping at the saucer of milk. Twenty minutes later, I was creeping silently toward him on hands and knees. What great fortune that he'd fallen asleep right next to the trap! As I wrapped my gloved hands around his middle, he came awake with a ferocious snarl, but I didn't stop. In one smooth motion, I lifted him a few inches off the wooden boards and into the trap. The door closed securely with a snap, as he reached out with both paws, claws fully extended. It was a close call.

I pulled the next piece of my arsenal from my pocket: a bottle of Nature's Rescue. I knew better than to try to give him some by mouth—I had another trick up my sleeve. Pouring a good quantity into one palm, I dipped the fingers of my other hand into it and flicked the droplets like gentle rain through the wire mesh of the cage onto his face. Having found their destination—the mucous membranes of his nose and eyes—they calmed him immediately, and he sat down on his good thigh.

From my vantage point I could see the abscess plainly. It was truly the worst I'd ever seen. The hole was easily a quarter inch in diameter and full of yellow-green discharge that drained sluggishly down his thigh; the edges of the wound looked dark red and puffy and had small cracks extending outward away from the hole. Big Head watched me with suspicious eyes but remained lying down.

Soon Marc joined me in the loft, and together we administered an injection of sedative through the wire mesh of the cage. It quickly took effect, and we pulled him out and flushed out the hole with hydrogen peroxide. Marc thought that the hole was big enough to allow the abscess to continue to drain on its own, so he chose not to surgically open it further.

"He's not going to like it, but you'll have to confine him to the tack room for a few days, so he can be kept warm and be given regular doses of Hepar sulph," Marc said when we were finished. "You'll also have to keep flushing this hole with peroxide every day until the discharges are gone and while it heals from the inside out." Big Head had a history of abscesses, but the first few times we had treated them with antibiotics, he had experienced allergic reactions. Although he was primarily a conventional vet, Marc agreed that Big Head responded well to homeopathic remedies, which, amazingly to him, worked on this kind of injury.

Over the next few days, I made regular visits to Big Head in the tack room. Four times a day, he got Hepar sulph in milk. Twice a day he was given a peroxide flush. He ate and slept and recuperated. As the abscess healed, he became easier to handle, but even in the beginning, after the first dose of Hepar sulph, which had reduced the pain to a level where he could be handled, he was willing to have me help him. Not once did he attempt to bite or scratch, and after the first two flushings with peroxide, he calmly let me wash out his wound while keeping a watchful eye on the proceedings.

By the fifth day of his confinement, the abscess was no longer draining, and I could see that the hole was rapidly filling in with healthy pink tissue. At this point, I reduced the Hepar sulph dosage to just twice a day, but still made many visits to keep him company and brought him freshly picked couch grass, such as he was used to eating in the surrounding fields. I also continued to superficially wash out the healing hole, to keep it open until it had entirely filled in with healthy tissue.

As the next few days passed, Big Head became more and more restless with his confinement. I took to playing with him during our visits. Clearly, with as much energy as he was displaying, he was nearly ready to be released. In just over a week of doses of Hepar sulph and peroxide flushes, the wound was covered in a healthy-looking scab. We had accomplished our goal of getting him on the mend, without bodily injury to any of his care-givers. I was happy to let him go, sure that he had much catching up to do in enforcing the perimeters of his domain.

At the barn door, where it opened onto the barnyard, Big Head stopped and sat down. He blinked in the bright spring sunlight and began to wash first one paw, then the other, in a lazy, nonchalant fashion. He turned, looked at me over his shoulder, his big yellow eyes half closed, and hissed at me. Then, without so much as a backward glance, he took off, padding confidently toward the field.

"You're welcome!" I shouted after him.

FIRST AID
AND CARE OF ABSCESSES

First thing to do: Flush out discharges with hydrogen peroxide, lightly salted water, or diluted calendula tincture.

Do not bandage; allow matter to surface and drain. All abscesses should heal from the inside out.

Daily: Keep opened and clean with hydrogen peroxide flushes, or lightly salted water, or diluted calendula tincture until healed.

Caution: Symptoms of tremors, convulsions, extreme lassitude, or fever may indicate serious infection that has spread to a vital organ (e.g., tooth abscess that spreads to the brain). *Seek veterinary attention immediately.*

HOMEOPATHY FOR ABSCESSES

Status critical: *Seek veterinary attention immediately.* Give doses (four pellets) at five- to ten-minute intervals en route to your veterinarian.

Status acute: After an initial dose (four pellets), doses may be repeated at one-hour intervals for up to four doses or until condition is relieved. In case of no relief, consult your veterinarian.

Status chronic: After an initial dose (four pellets), continue with two to four doses a day or until symptoms subside. If no relief is obtained, consult your veterinarian.

SYMPTOMS	REMEDY
Swollen, puffy, red, shiny surface; touch painful; desire for cold on area; animal is fretful, agitated, and thirstless	Apis
Abscesses that do not develop, crops of small abscesses that do not open, general or muscle soreness	Arnica
Recurrent and persistent boils painful to the touch and growing larger, slow draining, cracks in skin, intolerance of cold	Hepar sulph
Abscesses that develop from puncture wounds, wounded parts feel cold to the touch, resistance to warming from being covered, twitching of muscles near the wound, rheumatism beginning in lower limbs and ascending, cracking of joints	Ledum
Constantly moist skin with a foul odor, pimples/ulcers around abscess, abscessed teeth, excess salivation and mouth odor, symptoms worse from cold	Merc

CHAPTER 4

Accidents and Trauma

Here are five simple rules for helping in an accident:

1. If it's working, keep doing it.
2. If it's not working, stop.
3. If you don't know what you're doing, don't do anything.
4. When in doubt, call your veterinarian.
5. Call your veterinarian anyway.

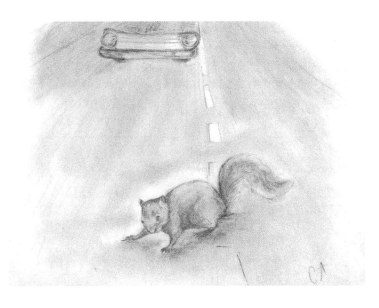

FIRST AID FOR ACCIDENTS AND TRAUMA

If bleeding is severe, apply direct pressure.

Firmly press a clean, dry pad or cloth to the wound (if you have
no pad, use your hand).

Keep pressing firmly enough to make bleeding stop. If pad
becomes soaked, put a second pad on top of first and press
harder. *Do not* remove first pad—this interrupts clotting action.

Keep pressing until bleeding stops or help is obtained.

Raise bleeding part higher than the heart to slow bleeding.

Treat for shock (cover the animal to retain body heat).

Seek veterinary attention immediately.

SEVERE WOUNDS

Do not try to clean.

Do not remove objects embedded in wound.

Do not remove the pressure pad.

MINOR WOUNDS

Wash out with warm water.

Apply a bandage.

Consult your veterinarian.

NOSE BLEEDING (CAN BE A SERIOUS CONDITION)

Keep the animal quiet.

Have animal sit and lean forward or lie down with head back and
raised.

Apply *direct pressure* by squeezing middle of the nose.

Apply cold compresses to head and face.

If bleeding does not stop in thirty minutes, consult your veterinarian.

HOMEOPATHY FOR ACCIDENTS AND TRAUMA

Status critical: *Seek veterinary attention immediately.* Give doses of four
pellets each at five- to ten-minute intervals en route to your veterinarian. If you see spurting bright red blood, it may be coming from

an artery; apply a pressure bandage and *seek veterinary attention immediately.*

Status acute: After an initial dose (four pellets), treatment may be repeated at fifteen-minute to half-hour intervals for up to four doses or until condition is relieved. If no relief is obtained, consult your veterinarian.

Status chronic: After an initial dose (four pellets), continue with two doses a day or until symptoms subside. If there is no relief, consult your veterinarian.

Symptoms	Remedy
Sudden and great fear, panic, and shock	Aconite (consider Nature's Rescue)
From falls and blows: soreness and bruising, hemorrhages under the skin, moderate shock	Arnica
Extreme trauma: stupor, collapse, or loss of consciousness; coldness of body, especially paws	Carbo veg
Trauma with bright red blood; fearful, jumpy; restless, fidgety	Phos
Overexertion or strains and sprains, joint and tendon injuries, continued morning stiffness	Rhus tox
Trauma with shock or fear	Nature's Rescue*

*Dilute four drops in an ounce of distilled water and give four drops of mixture on tongue or lips. Or hold open bottle under nose, as you would smelling salts. Repeat as needed.

CHAPTER 5

Back Injuries and Slipped Disks

Injuries to the spinal column and cord are usually very serious. Limping, numbness, inability to walk, or loss of bladder or bowel function (either retention or incontinence) are acute warning signs. Many animals who are unable to move as the result of such injuries are very frightened. Approach all injured animals with caution and remain calm so as not to frighten them even more. Your soothing voice and confident response will reassure both of you and assist you in getting to professional medical help as soon as possible.

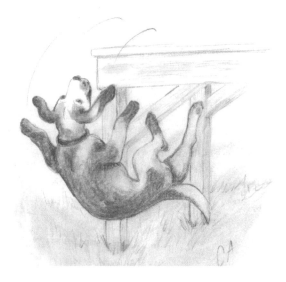

FIRST AID FOR
BACK INJURIES AND SLIPPED DISKS

Treat for shock (cover animal to retain body heat).

Treat as for injuries to skeletal system.

> *Do not* move animal unless necessary.
>
> *Seek veterinary attention immediately* and administer well-chosen remedies en route to your veterinary clinic.
>
> During transport, keep animal as immobile as possible. The use of a cardboard carton will prevent undue movement and give a sense of security to the animal (an open carton facilitates easier placement and removal than a commercial pet carrier).

HOMEOPATHY FOR
BACK INJURIES AND SLIPPED DISKS

Status critical: *Seek veterinary attention immediately.* Give doses of four pellets each at five- to ten-minute intervals en route to veterinarian.

Status acute: After an initial dose (four pellets), treatment may be repeated at one- to two-hour intervals for up to four doses or until relief is obtained. If there is no relief, consult your veterinarian.

Status chronic: After an initial dose (four pellets), continue with two doses a day or until symptoms subside. In case of no relief, consult your veterinarian.

SYMPTOMS	REMEDY
First remedy to consider for all cases of back injury; animal may be limping	Arnica
Violent, sudden, and intense pains; no thirst, anxiety, or fear; tottering gait, jerking limbs, spasm, and limping; cold extremities	Bell
Fractures to vertebra or tailbones (aids in healing bones)	Calc phos*
Injuries to the tail or toes, obvious nerve pain, symptoms worsen with touch, cold, dampness	Hyper

Symptoms	Remedy
Slipped disks with muscle spasms; numb legs, feet drag when walking; animal must sit up to turn over; irritable, resents touch[†]	Nux vom
Bruised bones with tendon/ligament involvement, legs give out easily, pain and stiffness of paws and joints, great restlessness	Ruta
Injuries penetrating to bones, injuries of sinews and tendons, nonunion of fractures, acute pain	Symph (use with Calc phos)

*A single daily dose is given until bones heal. Daily nutritional support consists of vitamin D (cod-liver oil, sunshine) and calcium (milk, yogurt, leafy greens). Avoid overexertion during healing.

[†]Continued numbness or lack of sensation in any limb may need veterinary attention.

CHAPTER 6

The Birthing Process

Usually our participation in the birthing process of any young animal is no more involved than witnessing the miracle of the continuation of life. Sometimes things seem to go wrong. In these instances, we are best advised to seek professional advice from our veterinarian. More often, a little help from us is welcomed and may make things easier. Homeopathy provides us with a gentle, nonintrusive way of giving assistance during this delicate event of life.

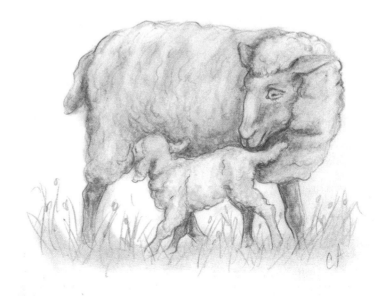

FIRST AID FOR THE BIRTHING PROCESS

General considerations for the well-being of mother and offspring are simple and stem from common sense. Birth is usually a natural process that takes place without the need for assistance, and unnecessary intervention may cause damage to the mother's reproductive tract or injury or death to the young.

Many animals, particularly mammals, will seek out and prepare their own private whelping, or delivery, place. All animals should be allowed to deliver their young in a clean, quiet, and familiar area where they will not be disturbed. Unfamiliar surroundings or the unwanted intrusion of strangers will often interfere with the birth process, milk letdown, or the mother's normal interaction with her young. For smaller animals, like cats, a cardboard box or carton big enough for the mother to lie down in makes an excellent whelping box. (An enclosed pen with low walls or a child's plastic wading pool can work well for dogs.) A towel folded tightly into a long roll and placed securely along the inside perimeter of the whelping box will keep the mother from rolling over onto her young and smothering them.

First-time mothers may be initially anxious, but this usually subsides very shortly. During labor, the cervix, vagina, and vulva (the external apparatus of the reproductive organs) become dilated to allow the passage of the young. Each offspring in a litter goes through its own birth process, and ample time should be allowed for each. Never pull the young from the birth canal; it may cause injury to the mother or young or both. The firstborn of a litter commonly takes longer than the rest, and the remaining young are born at shorter, regular intervals, each usually in its own placenta, or birth sack.

After the delivery of each newborn, the mother usually licks the infant's face, mouth, and nose to remove any remaining placenta that may impede breathing and any mucus from the respiratory tract. Licking also stimulates respiration and blood circulation. Always allow the mother time to attend to the young herself, but if she shows no interest, as is sometimes seen in inexperienced mothers, the infant may be assisted by the attendant.

To assist respiration:

> Elevate the infant's rear parts.
> For small animals, hold the head down and, while carefully supporting with a hand at the back of the neck, swing gently back and forth until the nostrils clear.

Rub gently but briskly to stimulate respiration.

If the birth is normal and the umbilical cord is not ruptured, leave it intact for five minutes. Contraction of the mother's uterus will force placental blood into the young, increasing its chances of survival. The mother will lick away any remaining placenta and mucus and will bite off the larger portion of the umbilical cord, leaving a stump. At this point, you may disinfect the end of the umbilical cord that is attached to the young with a cotton swab dipped in tincture of iodine or merthiolate. It is not necessary for the mother to consume the placenta, although it is natural for her to do so.

After the birth of each offspring, wait for the mother's mothering instinct to kick in. All young must be kept warm to prevent loss of body heat. The removal of the young from the delivery area after birth is usually not recommended, nor is picking them up or disturbing them (or the mother) during the birthing process. A mother that is giving birth for the first time may be anxious. Nervousness may be exhibited as ignoring the young or, conversely, as extreme overattentiveness, for example, continually licking them or biting and chewing at the umbilical cord. Such continuous unnecessary grooming may prevent the young from nursing or injure them. Gentle intervention may be necessary to prevent injury to the young; removing the harassed young may be necessary for a short interval of time, perhaps fifteen minutes. If this is required, be sure to keep the infant warm and quiet and replace the young in the delivery area as soon as the mother seems less anxious. Some new mothers, in their anxiety, may actually leave the delivery area. You may need to place the mother back in the delivery area and reassure her with soothing words.

It is very normal for all mothers, new or experienced, to rearrange each newborn in the delivery area after its birth, but afterward the mother should lie down and allow the infant to nurse. All the young should receive colostrum (the first, antibody-rich milk that the mother produces) as soon after birth as possible. Observe all young closely to see that they nurse shortly after birth. Occasionally, some young require assistance. With their heads higher than their tails, place their mouths carefully next to the teats or nipples, where they will have an opportunity to nurse. An infant that turns away from the nipple may be encouraged to nurse by gently rubbing his or her face into the nipple, both to arouse the suckling response and to stimulate milk flow.

All young should be monitored daily to make sure they are gaining weight and receiving enough milk. Daily weight gain in infants is also evidence that the mother is producing an adequate amount of milk. After the first day, all infants of any species should show signs of weight gain and growth. No weight gain or a loss of weight in any twenty-four-hour period should be immediately investigated by your veterinarian.

Postpartum, or after-birth, problems are easy to identify and usually encompass three areas: the placenta, the uterus, and the milk glands. Each young is normally delivered along with its own placenta. After each young is born, contractions will cease for a short time, until the next young enters the birth canal. Continued straining as if still in labor, after the birth of an infant, is the indication that a placenta has been retained. This condition is referred to as metritis and may lead to uterine infection if it is not corrected. In this event, do call your veterinarian, who will likely want to give an injection of oxytocin to cause expulsion of the retained placenta.

The uterus may also bleed excessively after the birth of one or more young. It will usually entail bleeding of large amounts of bright red blood. Small amounts of blood are not abnormal in any delivery, but watery blood that wets the delivery area or the mother's fur or that contains clots is worth noting. Pick a homeopathic remedy from the list given, but if, after a few doses, bleeding does not subside, call your veterinarian for assistance.

Failure of the milk glands to work properly may also be a postpartum problem. Refer to the section on mastitis (inflammation of the teats) and the chapter on homeopathy for orphaned puppies and kittens as well as the section that discusses substitute milk formulas for orphaned young.

HOMEOPATHY FOR THE BIRTHING PROCESS

Status critical: *Seek veterinary attention immediately.* Give doses of four pellets at five- to ten-minute intervals en route to the vet. Spurting of bright red blood after the birthing process is indicative of bleeding from an artery; apply a pressure bandage and *seek veterinary attention immediately.*

Status acute: After an initial dose (four pellets), treatment may be repeated at half-hour intervals for up to four doses or until condition is relieved. If no relief is obtained, consult your veterinarian.

Symptoms	Remedy
Difficult labor, observable bleeding, swelling and/or bruising	Arnica*
Excessive bleeding; watery, bright red blood; faint and anxious demeanor	Phosph
Moderate laboring pains, comforting seems welcomed	Puls†
Diminished secretion of milk, sluggish uterine bleeding, arrests flow of milk after weaning	Urt urens‡

*One dose is given after labor has stopped, followed by one or two doses daily for a few days, if needed.

†One dose is given after the first birth; repeat at half-hour intervals until last offspring is born.

‡Gently massage milk glands, if animal is willing. If milk does not flow after several doses, use milk formula substitute (see Appendix) and consult your veterinarian for care of the mother. See also chapter 26 (Mastitis) and chapter 27 (Orphaned Kittens and Puppies).

CHAPTER 7

Bites from Animals

Sometimes cute and cuddly and at other times stalking ferociously in their play and interactions with other animals, our animal companions are a continual delight and surprise to us, their moods and inner landscape always changing. No matter how domestic or docile we think our animal friends are, they are animals. They do sometimes fight and quarrel, expressing their animal nature in its most pure and savage form: with their teeth and claws. Often, we see only the aftermath of their unfettered excursions into their wild natures. But bites and gashes need not be alarming to us if we know what to do ahead of time.

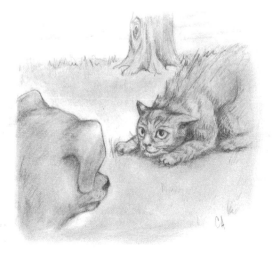

THAT'S MY JAKE

I stood at the window in the back hall of the farmhouse and looked out on a blustery autumn day. The wind lifted leaves high in the air and swept them still further upward in small tornadoes of current. Jake should be out there playing; chasing leaves was his favorite pastime next to investigating beetles. But he was nowhere to be seen. I opened the door and went out to call him.

In response to my voice, I heard a plaintive wail coming from the back end of the flower garden. It was Jake, and I rushed past the rosebushes and azaleas. He was hunched up behind two short rows of marigolds, lying on his side with his left paw stretched out painfully on the ground. Even before I reached him, I could see how he held his paw away from him and how he shivered with a chill. I scooped him into my arms, no small feat, for Jake was a huge tomcat weighing in at just under seventeen pounds.

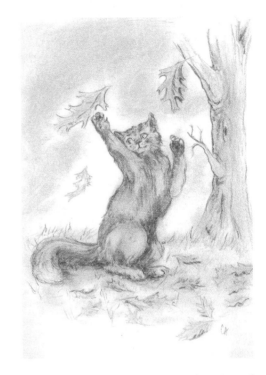

In the kitchen, I filled the sink with warm water and placed a towel on the counter at the edge of the sink. Once Jake was positioned on the towel, I took his paw in my hand and placed it in the water to soak for a few minutes. He's such a character, my Jake. He sat there watching, looking at his paw dangling in the water. After a few minutes, he pulled his paw out and held it up in front of his chest. He was letting me know that it still hurt. Since the fur was very wet and no longer fluffy, I could easily see the deep puncture wound just below the first joint of his front paw. It was a neat hole with smooth edges, a perfectly round circle, one sixteenth of an inch in diameter. It was a bite, and a deep one, too—probably from another cat. Feeling fortunate that I have always been conscientious about our animal companions' immunizations, I had no fear of contagious diseases. But a homeopathic remedy would hasten healing of this traumatic injury; with the right one, given at correct intervals, Jake should be chasing leaves before the next autumn rainstorm.

I placed him in a cushioned wicker chair in the kitchen. As I lifted him, I noticed that his body felt very cold to my touch, so I covered him with a small blanket that was draped over the back of the chair. As I suspected, he at once shrugged off the blanket. This was an important clue that Ledum palustre was the remedy he needed. The typical animal needing Ledum is very chilled, sometimes almost shivering, yet he or she will resist all attempts to be warmed or covered.

On my way to the hall closet to get our household homeopathic kit, I gave the thermostat dial a twist. To turn on the oil furnace on such a sunny autumn day was a luxury. Had I not been in such a hurry, I might have made a small fire in the kitchen woodstove as well, but getting Jake warmed was a priority, and I had no time to be feeding kindling and oak knots into the firebox.

Soon I returned with the bottle of Ledum 30c. Jake was lying on top of the blanket and chewing at his injured paw as though it itched—another Ledum symptom. Jake is an independent cat. Although he will often reach out and tap me on the shoulder with his paw if he thinks he should be getting more attention than I am giving him, he generally does not like fuss and caresses to an extreme. He is the same way about taking his remedies and resents having his mouth opened to have the pillules placed there. Fortunately, homeopathic remedies can be dissolved in milk, since the pillules are made from a base of milk sugar. And, very fortunately, Jake really likes milk and will lap his remedy up as long as he doesn't see me putting the pillules in it.

I poured four pillules of Ledum 30c into a small saucer, without touching them, and then added about a tablespoon of milk from the refrigerator. After stirring with a spoon for a minute or so, until they were dissolved, I placed the saucer on the chair within easy reach. Seeing the milk, Jake forgot all about his itchy paw.

He lapped the milk up quickly and then settled in for a thorough cleanup, beginning with his whiskers and face and finishing with both front paws. Soon he was curled up in the chair fast asleep.

When he awoke almost an hour later, he jumped down from the wicker chair, using both front feet to execute his landing maneuver. Then, after ravaging the salmon, rice, and vegetables in his bowl, he returned to his chair for another nap. During the late afternoon and again just before bedtime, I gave him two more single doses of Ledum. From the look of him after his first nap, I felt that he was well on his way to mending. Sure enough, the next morning he was out in the garden again, stalking soaring leaves. I watched him as he played, frivolous and frisky as a kitten. I wasn't surprised when, a short while later, the sky grayed and a few raindrops began to fall.

FIRST AID FOR BITES FROM ANIMALS

SEVERE ANIMAL BITES

If bleeding is severe, *apply direct pressure.*

> Firmly press a clean, thick, dry pad or cloth to the wound (if you have no pad, use your hand).
>
> Keep pressing firmly enough to make the bleeding stop. If pad becomes soaked, put a second pad on top of the first, and press harder. *Do not* remove first pad—this interrupts clotting action.
>
> Keep pressing until bleeding stops or help is obtained.
>
> Raise bleeding part higher than the heart to slow bleeding.

Treat for shock (cover the animal to retain body heat).

Immediate care of bite wounds

> *Do not* try to clean.
>
> *Do not* remove objects embedded in wound.
>
> *Do not* remove the pressure pad.
>
> *Seek veterinary attention immediately.*

MINOR ANIMAL BITES

Wash with soap and water.

> Soak daily in hydrogen peroxide, salty water, or diluted calendula tincture to keep wound clean and open. Allow all punctures to heal from the inside out.

Loosely bandage, if necessary.

> Choose a homeopathic remedy from the list given.

HOMEOPATHY FOR BITES FROM ANIMALS

Status critical (snakebites, scorpion stings): *Seek veterinary attention immediately.* Give doses of four pellets at five- to ten-minute intervals en route to veterinarian.

Status acute: After an initial dose (four pellets), treatment may be repeated at fifteen-minute to half-hour intervals for up to four doses. *Seek veterinary attention immediately.*

Status chronic: After an initial dose (four pellets), continue with two doses a day or until symptoms subside. If there is no relief, consult your veterinarian.

SYMPTOMS	REMEDY
First remedy to consider; pain, inflammation, and fear; follow with any remedy on this list	Aconite (consider Nature's Rescue)
Minor bites with bruising and pain; severe and dirty bites; redness, swelling, heat	Arnica Hepar sulph
Painful puncture bites with nerve pain, threatened tetanus	Hyper
Puncture bites; snakebites, scorpion stings; purple or blue discoloration; swelling and festering	Lach
Deep puncture bites; coldness of body, but aversion to warming; bites become itchy	Ledum
Bites with shock or fear	Nature's Rescue*

*Dilute four drops in an ounce of distilled water and give four drops of mixture on tongue or lips. Or hold open bottle under nose, as you would with smelling salts. Repeat as needed. In cases of bites accompanied by shock, *seek veterinary attention immediately.*

CHAPTER 8
Bleeding

Seeing our beloved animal companion bleeding, whether copiously or slightly, causes most of us to experience a feeling of great alarm. A cool head, deep breathing, and a firm resolve are our best tools in such an emergency. With these measures in place, we can then assess the situation and do the things that need to be done. Our calmness and self-assurance will help our animal companions feel confident in our ministrations. Believe that you can make a difference, and you can.

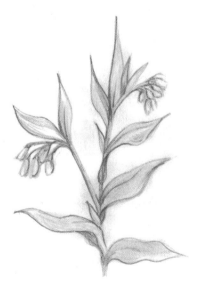

Comfrey

A CASE OF PHOSPHORUS FOR BLEEDING

I didn't see the truck run the red light. The impact was sudden and violent and sent my compact sedan flying across the intersection, where we struck a tree with a sickening jolt. Glass was flying everywhere; it sprayed across my lap, and, out of the corner of my eye, I saw a ragged chunk of the windshield soar past my shoulder into the backseat, where Caleb, my German shepherd, had been sitting moments before.

When stillness reigned once again, I turned slowly to see if he was all right. I couldn't see him on the seat, and with rising panic I brushed glass off my lap and struggled to raise up just enough to look behind the front seat. He was there on the floor, in a huddled heap, trying, I saw with relief, to gain his footing. He was alive.

Suddenly people were rushing around outside the car. "Don't move," I heard an unfamiliar voice say. I took a shaky breath and turned back around. Within moments, with the help of two people who had stopped, my dog and I were both out of the car and sitting shakily on the curb. I put my arm around Caleb and held him tightly to me. Something sticky and wet was flowing onto my arm. I looked down and saw a huge gash on his shoulder; the windshield fragment had found a target, and a yielding one, too. He was bleeding copiously and seemed wobbly and dazed.

Shock, I thought. Apply a pressure bandage; stop the blood flow. Grateful that I had thought to put a clean bandana in my jeans' pocket that morning, I folded it somewhat smaller and pressed it firmly to the gash. It was immediately soaked through, and I hadn't another; I wasn't even wearing a light jacket, despite the cool autumn day. With my free hand, I reached down and pulled the bottom of my T-shirt free from the waistband of my jeans. Taking a fold in my hand, I brought it to my mouth and chewed a small hole in the fabric—just enough to get a tear started. As I pulled, Caleb slumped forward into my lap; he was growing weak from so much blood loss. I had to hurry. I had to reach around my back to tear the cloth loose, but I managed to rip off quite a large portion. Once I had freed it, I bunched the cloth in my fist and placed it over the first bandage and pressed harder.

I knew not to remove the first layer of bandage; that would only interrupt the clotting action that had already begun. As I held the scrap of cloth in place, I spoke softly to Caleb, reassuring him that everything was going to be fine. The sound of my voice also reassured me and brought the owner of the unfamiliar voice over to us.

"How are you doing?" the elderly gentleman said with concern. "I feel pretty much all right," I answered. "But my dog is bleeding a lot. Would you see if you could find a handkerchief and something to cover him, so he won't go into shock? I need to keep his body heat in; he's lost a lot of blood. Also, there's a small first-aid kit in the glove compartment of my car. Would you get that, please? It's really important."

The man looked around for something to give me. He, too, was dressed lightly for the day, without even a sweater. He strode off toward his own car and came back a moment later with a thick newspaper, which he spread over Caleb, tucking the edges under him. I noted that the bleeding had nearly stopped; the crumpled scrap of T-shirt under my hand was still mostly dry. As much as I wanted to, I resisted the impulse to lift up the bandage and have a look at the extent of the wound. The pressure bandage mustn't be removed until we got to the veterinary clinic. I hoped that would be very soon.

In another minute the elderly man came back with the small homeopathic kit that I keep in my car. I thanked him as I opened it with my free hand and took out the small vial of Phosphorus 30c. I looked down at Caleb. He was panting slightly, his eyes closed, still slumped in my arms.

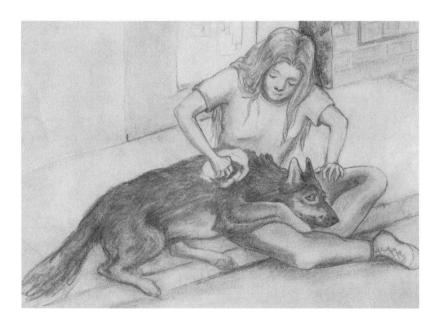

Aconitum napellus, commonly called Aconite, for shock would be helpful, too, I decided. Together we placed four pillules of Phosphorus in Caleb's right cheek pouch and four pillules of Aconite in his left cheek pouch. Unconventional? Sure, but this was no ordinary situation.

"I came as quickly as I heard," a familiar voice sounded behind me. "Sarah from across the street saw the accident and drove straight to our house to tell me." I looked up to see the concerned face of my husband looking into my own. "Are you both okay?" he asked. I nodded. "I think we're both all right, but we've got to get him to Marc's clinic. Now. I think this gash is going to need quite a few stitches. But the bleeding seems to have stopped; that's the good thing."

Angus helped us both into the backseat of his station wagon and placed the car blanket over us lovingly, tenderly tucking us in for the short ride ahead. Everything was going to be fine, I thought, as I looked at Caleb lying on the seat beside me. He stirred under my hand, which was still pressing the bandage to his shoulder, and looked up confidently into my eyes. We were going to be all right. I took his paw in my free hand and gave it a gentle squeeze. In response, he flexed his toes in the palm of my hand as if to squeeze back. Even Caleb knew we were going to be fine.

FIRST AID FOR BLEEDING

Severe bleeding must be controlled.

If bleeding is severe, *apply direct pressure.*

> Firmly press a clean, thick, dry pad or cloth to the wound (if no pad is available, use your hand).
>
> Keep pressing firmly enough to make the bleeding stop. If pad becomes soaked, put a second pad on top of the first and press harder. *Do not* remove first pad—this interrupts clotting action.
>
> Keep pressing until bleeding stops or help is obtained.
>
> Raise the bleeding part higher than the heart to slow bleeding.

Treat for shock (cover the animal to retain body heat).

Seek veterinary attention immediately.

BAD WOUNDS

> *Do not* try to clean it.
>
> *Do not* remove objects embedded in wound.

Treat for bleeding.

Do not remove the pressure pad.

Treat for shock (cover animal to retain body heat).

Seek veterinary attention immediately.

MINOR CUTS AND WOUNDS

Wash out with warm water.

Apply a bandage.

Consult your veterinarian.

NOSE BLEEDING (MAY BE A SERIOUS CONDITION)

Keep the animal quiet.

Have the animal sit and lean forward or lie down with head back and raised.

Apply *direct pressure* by squeezing middle of the nose.

Apply cold compresses to head and face.

If bleeding does not stop in thirty minutes, consult your veterinarian.

HOMEOPATHY FOR BLEEDING

Status critical: *Seek veterinary attention immediately.* Give doses of four pellets at five- to ten-minute intervals en route to your veterinarian. Bright red spurting blood or bleeding that lasts more than fifteen minutes may be coming from an artery; apply a pressure bandage en route to your veterinarian.

Status acute: After an initial dose (four pellets), treatment may be repeated at fifteen-minute intervals for another couple of doses. If treatment gives no relief, *seek veterinary attention immediately.*

Status chronic: After an initial dose (four pellets), continue with a dose or two or until symptoms subside. If no relief is obtained, *seek veterinary attention immediately.*

SYMPTOMS	REMEDY
Bleeding with signs of shock; bright red blood; anxiety, faintness	Aconite (consider Nature's Rescue)
Bleeding from a blow, blunt trauma	Arnica

Symptoms	Remedy
Bleeding with collapse	Carbo veg
Copious bleeding; watery, bright red blood	Phosph
Any bleeding with shock or fear	Nature's Rescue*

*Dilute four drops in an ounce of distilled water and give four drops of mixture on tongue or lips. Or hold open bottle under the nose, as you would with smelling salts. Repeat as needed. If bleeding is accompanied by shock, *seek veterinary attention immediately.*

CHAPTER 9

Bone Injuries

Accidents resulting in bone injuries, like fractures (broken bones), dislocations, and bruised bones, are fortunately uncommon among animals. Most cases are the result of animals' being struck down by cars or trucks, and they less frequently stem from falls from heights. Calm reassurance of your animal companion, correct handling, and rapid transport to a veterinary facility are the keys to a successful outcome. This may be a situation in which everyone involved will benefit from a few drops of Nature's Rescue.

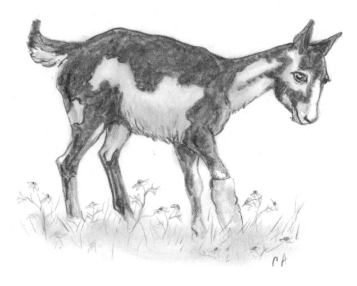

FIRST AID FOR BONE INJURIES

Treat fractures and dislocations in the same way.

Do not move the animal unless absolutely necessary.

In all cases treat the most serious injury first.

Control bleeding with *gentle direct pressure.*

Gently press a clean, thick, dry pad or cloth to the wound (if you have no pad, use your hand).

Keep pressing gently. If the pad becomes soaked, put a second pad on top of the first. *Do not* remove first pad—this interrupts clotting action.

If bleeding continues, apply additional padding.

Raise the bleeding part higher than the heart, to slow bleeding.

Treat for shock (cover the animal to retain body heat).

Treat bone injury

Apply a bandage to the fracture very loosely, and tape gently into place. *Do not* apply slings or splints unless you are trained to do so.

Do not touch or wash. Bone injuries that pierce skin become infected easily.

Do not disturb bones or bone chips. If bits of bone or skin have become detached, place in a clean, airtight plastic bag and take with the animal to your veterinarian (they may be reattached).

Try to keep animal immobilized en route to your veterinarian.

Seek veterinary attention immediately.

HOMEOPATHY FOR BONE INJURIES

Status critical: *Seek veterinary attention immediately.* Give doses of four pellets at five- to ten-minute intervals en route to your veterinarian.

Status acute: After an initial dose (four pellets), treatment may be repeated at fifteen-minute to half-hour intervals for up to four doses or until relief is obtained. If there is no relief, consult your veterinarian.

Status chronic: After an initial dose (four pellets), continue with two doses a day for one week or until symptoms subside. If there is no relief, consult your veterinarian.

Symptoms	Remedy
First remedy to consider; shock (usually accompanies pain); trauma, faintness	Aconite (consider Nature's Rescue)
General pain of bone injuries	Arnica
Aids in healing fractures after break has been set and cast	Calc phos*
After fractures heal: lingering stiffness, especially on rising in the morning	Rhus tox
Bone breaks with joint and tendon involvement, pain in bones and surrounding structures, nonunion or slow-healing fractures, wounds penetrating to bone surface	Symph
Any trauma or bone injury with shock or fear	Nature's Rescue[†]

*Administer a single daily dose until bones heal. For daily nutritional support give vitamin D (cod-liver oil, sunshine) and calcium (milk, yogurt, leafy greens). Avoid overexertion during healing.

[†]Dilute four drops in an ounce of distilled water and give four drops of mixture on tongue or lips. Or hold open bottle under the nose, as you would with smelling salts. Repeat as needed. Any trauma accompanied by shock, *seek veterinary attention immediately.*

CHAPTER 10

Bruises

Whether we have exuberant puppies or kittens full of enthusiastic wonder or active older animals, bumps, bruises, and other minor injuries do happen occasionally and may seem more serious than they really are. Once you have checked with your veterinarian to be sure that no serious injury has been sustained by your animal companion, there is a great deal that homeopathy can do to relieve minor discomfort and facilitate full, rapid healing. In the event that multiple symptoms are present, such as in the case of an accident that results in cuts, a sprain, and bruising, more than

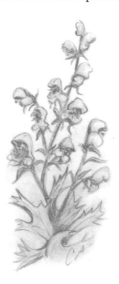

Monkshood

one remedy may be used at once. Remedies may also be given in succession to address all symptoms arising from a minor injury.

FIRST AID FOR BRUISES

Bruises are the result of blunt trauma, usually to muscle tissues and sometimes to bones. Swelling and blue or purple discolorations on the skin are due to the hemorrhaging of blood under the surface of the skin. Cold compresses may relieve discomfort, and gentle rubbing may also give relief. No one knows your animal companion better than you! Follow his or her lead and do only that which he or she indicates is comfortable and helpful. Never force animals to tolerate massage or a cold pack if they resist such aid.

Consult your veterinarian. If simple bruising is the only symptom, with no other complications, employ one or both of the following therapies—but only if your animal companion does not resist.

Apply cold compresses to the bruised area three or four times a day until discomfort subsides.

Very gently massage the affected area.

Never exercise or work an animal that is bruised. *Rest and relaxation are a necessary part of healing.*

HOMEOPATHY FOR BRUISES

Status critical: *Seek veterinary attention immediately.* Give doses of four pellets at five- to ten-minute intervals en route to your veterinarian.

Status acute: After an initial dose (four pellets), dosage may be repeated at one- to two-hour intervals for up to four doses or until condition is relieved. If there is no relief, consult your veterinarian.

Status chronic: After an initial dose (four pellets), continue with two doses a day or until symptoms subside. If no relief is obtained, consult your veterinarian.

Symptoms	Remedy
First remedy to consider, trauma with shock or fear, bruising and numbness of affected area, great fear and anxiety	Aconite (consider Nature's Rescue)
Classic remedy for all bruises and blows with pain, soreness, lameness, stiffness, swelling with purple discoloration; indifference to consolation; fear of touch or approach; desire to be left alone	Arnica
Trauma with shock or fear	Nature's Rescue*

*Dilute four drops in an ounce of distilled water and give four drops of mixture on tongue or lips. Or hold open bottle under the nose, as you would with smelling salts. Repeat as needed. Any trauma accompanied by shock, *seek veterinary attention immediately.*

CHAPTER 11

Burns and Scalds

There is no health emergency quite as alarming as a burn or scald to an animal. Quite often, the animal's initial reaction to such a painful injury is fear and withdrawal. Shock may also be present owing to the intensity of pain. As stewards of the animals in our lives, our first responsibility is to provide a safe environment in which accidents are unlikely to happen in the first place. We all do the best we can. However, in the event that your animal companion sustains a serious burn, this is one first-aid section you'll be glad you read ahead of time.

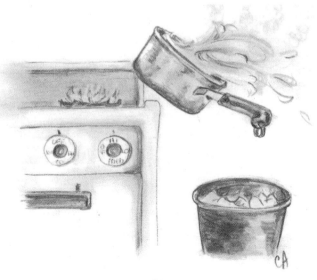

IN A HURRY TO SLOW DOWN

Jeanette and I had gone into the far reaches of rural Maine to work as summer volunteers for the Moosewood Wildlife Refuge. We were excited about spending eight weeks in an unspoiled wilderness area and eager to learn about the indigenous animal and plant life of Maine, in an environment that was as natural and wild as any left in North America. The only hitch was that our accommodations were not provided, and it was left to us to find a place to rent for the two months we would be there, a place that would permit us to keep our three cats.

Our search ended on our second day when we found a small trailer for rent, for a fee that seemed almost too good to be true. During the second week in our new temporary home, we found out why the rent was so cheap: the hot-water heater gave its last gallon of tepid water (after what I suspect was many years of laborious service to a steady stream of tenants), and one morning at 2 A.M. the refrigerator gave a loud gasp that ended in a jolting clunking noise, at which point the motor in the bottom came to its final resting place—on the floor.

But we were there to enjoy the wilderness, and enjoy it we would. Undaunted that it had followed us indoors, we set about living life the old-fashioned way. After grueling days following moose through bogs and sitting patiently in the splendor of creek banks to count beaver, we carried ice home to be placed in what was now an old-fashioned icebox. And in the early evenings, in great need of rejuvenating soaks, we heated huge kettles of water on the kitchen stove and carried them down the trailer hall to fill the bathtub.

It was on one of these evenings that the accident happened. Jeanette, carefully carrying a fresh kettle of nearly boiling water, was met by Duffy, her yellow tiger Persian, who had streaked out into the hall to ravish her ankles in a playful mood. Startled and wincing from the shock of sharp claws on bare skin, Jeanette lost her grip on the kettle, and the unfortunate Duffy was drenched from his ears downward in very hot water. I had been sitting in a visually advantageous place in the living room and watched with horror as the entire scene unfolded in a matter of seconds.

Almost without thinking, I was up and out of my chair and racing toward them. Duffy, in a typical fright response, was already fleeing down the hall and, fortunately for him, in my direction. As I passed him in my flight toward the bathroom, I scooped him into my arms like a quarterback recapturing a football on the spin. Our destination was the bathtub, which was half full of cold water, waiting to be filled to the top with the kettles of hot water.

He didn't resist being picked up; as soon as I touched him, he went limp. Even before I had taken two running steps with him in my arms, the thick sleeves of my sweatshirt were soaked with burning hot water. I took the last two feet toward the tub in a leap, stopping only because my knees met the ceramic edge with a painful thump.

I quickly lowered him into the cold water. He still didn't resist, but floated there on his back with my arms under him. He looked up into my eyes, his eyes reflecting fear, pain, and anguish. I spoke in what I hoped was a reassuring tone, telling him that he was going to be all right. Jeanette was suddenly behind me. Without saying a word, she turned on the cold-water

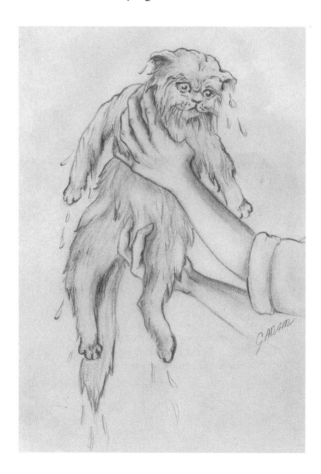

tap, and a gentle stream of cold water flowed into the half-full tub. At once I could feel through my soaked sleeves that the water temperature dropped even further.

When Duffy began to struggle a few minutes later, I thought that he had had enough. We took him, loosely wrapped in a towel, to Jeanette's bed to examine the extent of the burns. Aside from a blister on the upper edge of one ear and a red, shiny patch at the base of his spine where it met his tail and where the fur was naturally thin, he seemed to not be too severely burned. The remainder of his body had been mildly burned, and the skin was red and slightly inflamed, but, luckily for him, his heavy fur had acted as insulation against the brunt of most of the hot water. When I touched various parts of his back, thighs, and shoulders, he winced, and I noted that he felt warm. At this point, he began to resist being touched anywhere on his body; he seemed to hurt all over. Since the burns were blistering and he was extremely sensitive to touch, I thought that he was a good candidate for Apis mellifica 30c. But first, because he had been through a shocking ordeal and was obviously restless, I believed he would be greatly helped by a dose of Aconite 30c.

Jeanette was one step ahead of me. With a deft motion she lifted Duffy's lip and poured four pillules of Aconite into the space between his cheek and gum. We waited for the remedy to work. He calmed perceptibly within a few minutes but then became restless again, shifting first to one side, then another. Jeanette gave him another dose of Aconite, and within minutes Duffy was calm again.

"I think we should go with the Apis now. The blister on his ear is puffing rapidly, and so is the bare patch at the base of his tail." Jeanette's voice sounded tense and worried. I quickly tried to put things in perspective. "I don't know anyone who takes better care of their cats than you, Jeanette. I remember when Jane had been missing for five hours last fall. You stayed out all night until you found her. No one else would ever have thought to look in that blocked storm drain. And after the rain that came the next day, well, you obviously saved her life. This wasn't your fault. You couldn't have known that Duffy was planning a surprise ambush; I was watching, and it happened so quickly that had I been right there, I wouldn't have been able to prevent it."

Jeanette attempted a brave smile. "I know it's not my fault. I just feel so bad that it happened. Here, I've got the Apis. I just hope this will help." As with the Aconite, Jeanette gave Duffy a dose. When she was finished, she stroked Duffy's salmon-colored nose. I was immensely thankful that his face, mouth, and eyes had been spared.

My first reaction upon reaching the bathtub was to ask Jeanette to bring ice to put into the water. But I remembered my first-aid course: never use ice on burns; it can further damage injured skin. Because the two most severe burns were blistered (the second layer of tissue having been damaged), they were categorized as second-degree burns. These, according to what I had learned, could be bandaged, but I doubted that Duffy would leave the gauze and tape alone. I also knew from the same course that burns must have air to heal, and I decided that leaving them uncovered was the best idea. As for the rest of his burned skin, it was red and mildly inflamed, indicative of first-degree burns. These would heal more rapidly than his ear and the base of his tail, but he would need rest, extra fluids, and peace and quiet.

I decided to confine him to Jeanette's bedroom for the next few days and set about arranging his litter box and food bowls in the room. I replaced the water in his water bowl with electrolyte solution to make sure that he remained hydrated. Then I got a footstool from the living room and placed it at the foot of the bed, so that he could get up and down comfortably without having to stretch out his body (and his skin), as cats do when they leap up onto surfaces higher than the floor. This done, I went out to the hall to clean up the accident scene.

The next day, when I looked in on him, Duffy seemed much better. He was sitting on the chest of drawers looking out the window. Jeanette had given him a second dose of Apis before bedtime the night before. Already the redness and inflammation over most of his body looked to be well on its way to being healed. And the blisters on his ear and lower back had lost their puffiness; most of the fluid had been reabsorbed by his body. His mental state was relaxed as well; he greeted my arrival with his usual trill and seemed happy to see me.

We continued administering Apis 30c for the next four days. Initially, we gave it to him four times a day. When the pace of the healing picked up, we reduced the frequency of doses to twice a day. By the fifth day, the worst burns were almost healed, and Duffy was freed from his confinement.

Late that evening, after having filled the bath with hot water, Jeanette opened the door to my bedroom, where each evening all three cats waited patiently—and safely—for the nightly ritual to be completed. Jane came out first, followed swiftly by Jiggles. A few minutes later, from my vantage point in the living room, I peered up over the top of the newspaper to see a wee bit of salmon-colored nose appear cat level at the edge of the door casing. It was followed by Duffy's head. Yellow eyes looked up the hallway, then down the hallway. Seeing the coast was clear, he scrabbled at the carpeting with his hind claws, found a solid purchase, and was off like a flash chasing the other cats. With a hearty chuckle, I returned to the article I had been reading in the newspaper. It was an interview with a southern Maine veterinarian who had begun using homeopathic remedies in his practice. Now that was news worth printing.

FIRST AID FOR BURNS AND SCALDS

All burns need air to heal. *Never* use ice. Use cold water only. Submerge or rinse in cold water.

First thing to do: Examine the extent of the burn. Look under the fur. If the skin is intact, apply or submerge in cold water. Never use ice.

Burns are categorized by depth. First-degree burns are superficial, second-degree burns extend to the middle-layer of the skin, and third-degree burns are the deepest.

First-degree burns: superficial, stemming from minor sunburns or hot liquids, red and slightly swollen.

Second-degree burns: affecting middle skin layer, from deep sunburns or flash burns from chemicals, blistered and wet-looking.

Third-degree burns: involving the deepest skin destruction, white and puffy or charred and black.

FIRST- AND SECOND-DEGREE BURNS

Submerge or rinse with cold water or apply a clean cloth soaked in cold water.

If blisters are closed, apply a clean, dry bandage.

If blisters are open, *do not* cover.

Do not break blisters open. *Do not* peel skin.

Let heal naturally.

If blister is large or does not heal, consult your veterinarian.

THIRD-DEGREE BURNS

Do not move the animal unless necessary.

Do not immerse in cold water.

Treat for shock (cover animal to retain body heat).

Apply a clean, thick, dry dressing (don't wrap, just cover).

Do not remove burned skin or charred material.

Seek veterinary attention immediately.

CHEMICAL BURNS TO SKIN (ODORS AND BLISTERING)

Get chemical off skin!

Remove any fabric and collar.

Wet chemicals: Rinse with *lots* of lukewarm water.

Dry chemicals: Brush off as completely as possible without
    spreading or pushing deeper, then rinse with lukewarm water.

Seek veterinary attention immediately.

HOMEOPATHY FOR BURNS AND SCALDS

Status critical: *Seek veterinary attention immediately.* Give doses of four
    pellets at five- to ten-minute intervals en route to your veterinar-
    ian.

Status acute: After an initial dose (four pellets), treatment may be
    repeated at half-hour intervals for up to four doses or until condi-
    tion is relieved. If no relief is obtained, consult your veterinarian.

Status chronic: After an initial dose (four pellets), continue with two
    doses a day or until symptoms subside. If condition is not relieved,
    consult your veterinarian.

SYMPTOMS	REMEDY
Always given first; extreme pain with shock; intolerable pain; restless tossing, extreme fear	Aconite (consider Nature's Rescue)

Symptoms	Remedy
Burns that puff up suddenly, fluid collecting under the skin, animal cannot bear touch	Apis
Blistered burns and scalds, raw and smarting; better from cold, but cold causes more inflammation; extreme restlessness	Canth
Burns with shock or fear	Nature's Rescue*

*Dilute four drops in an ounce of distilled water and give four drops of mixture on tongue or lips. Or hold open bottle under the nose, as you would with smelling salts. Repeat as needed. Any burns accompanied by shock, *seek veterinary attention immediately.*

CHAPTER 12

Car Sickness and Motion Sickness

The majority of us have too much to do in too little time. Our vehicles have become indispensable parts of our lives and make us immediately able to accomplish all the tasks we have to do on a daily basis. But what is a quick trip for us can be a very unpleasant event for our dog or cat. If our animals are plagued by vomiting, diarrhea, or physical discomfort when riding in our car or truck, it can end up being unpleasant for everyone. Homeopathic remedies do offer a solution, and all can be well. Going for a ride can be fun for everyone.

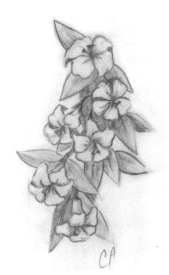

Yellow Jasmine

I LOVE YOU TOO

My sister, Karen, was on the phone. She had adopted a new dog from her local shelter, a rottweiler, two years old and very happy with her new home. Shawna they called her, and her disposition was as soft as the sound of her name. Shawna loved to go for rides in the car, anywhere and with any member of the family. My sister's family is one of those modern-day families—always on their way somewhere else and, it seems, always in the car. The problem was that although Shawna loved to go in the car, because going in the car meant being with her family, the motion always made her sick.

"Explain her symptoms exactly," I asked Karen, pressing for further details. "I think she gets carsick. At first she is restless; then she starts yawning, panting, and drooling. Sometimes she loses control of her bladder or bowel. Then she vomits all over the car. Once she even fainted. Boy, was I scared when that happened.

"I used to get sick riding in the car when I was little, too. Remember? It always helped me to have the window open so I could breathe fresh air, but that doesn't seem to help Shawna. In fact, if the air is cold, it seems to make her worse. Afterward, when we get where we're going, she won't drink water or eat anything for hours and hours. Even though I try to make her drink some water, she absolutely refuses.

"Bill just got his new car, and he's kind of annoyed that he's had to line

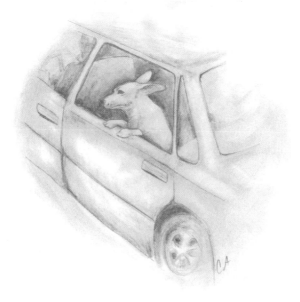

the whole backseat and floor with plastic and newspapers. He's not mad; none of us is. We just feel so bad for her."

"What about leaving her home some of the time?" I suggested hopefully.

"We can sometimes. But we want her to bond with us, and we want her to be able to go with us a lot. You know how we are—always on the go. I couldn't bear for her to be alone too much. She's really great; she's really a people dog. Just what we wanted. Is there anything we can do or anything we can give her? Something natural?"

I suggested Cocculus indicus 30c, one or two doses at half-hour intervals before the trip. "You can also repeat one or two doses if the symptoms appear en route. And give up on the idea that she should drink water after she vomits. By her adamant refusal to do so, she's telling you that she really can't."

"I'll give it a try!" Karen said enthusiastically.

"Call me in a few days and let me know how it's going, okay?"

"All right. I love you," she said, with an expectant lilt in her voice.

"I love you too," I said, chuckling, completing our telephone ritual.

I was at work when she called, but she left a message on my answering machine. I listened smiling. "How did you know?" her voice came through the speaker. "The first time, we gave it to her twice before we left. We'd gone about ten miles, and I was watching her in the rearview mirror and saw her panting. When I got to a rest stop I gave her some more, and in just a few minutes she looked fine again. When we arrived at Bill's Mom's house, she was fine. I can't believe how fast the Cocculus worked! Bill's really happy, too. He can't wait to take all the newspaper out of his car."

There was a pause. "I love you," she said, with that expectant high note at the end. There was a click, followed by a dial tone and the final beep, signaling the end of the message.

"I love you too," I said to the machine.

FIRST AID FOR CAR SICKNESS AND MOTION SICKNESS

COMMON INDICATIONS OF CAR OR MOTION SICKNESS
Pacing and whining
Panting, drooling, and repeated swallowing

Lying down on the floor of the vehicle (usually due to dizziness)

These symptoms escalate to dizziness, nausea, vomiting and/or diarrhea, followed by lack of thirst and/or appetite.

Repeated episodes may result in reluctance to get into a vehicle
(both your animal's reluctance and yours!).

WHAT TO DO

If car or motion sickness is impending or in progress

Stop the vehicle.

Take your animal out of the vehicle for fresh air and walk him or
her away from exhaust fumes. If cats are confined in a transport carrier, remove the carrier to an area of fresh air, with the
cat remaining inside.

Offer fresh water, but do not force the animal to drink.

Before returning the animal to the vehicle, clean up any accidents. If you have been prepared and have lined the car floor
or transport carrier with newspaper or plastic, this will be easier than cleaning carpeting.

Choose from the homeopathic remedies listed and follow instructions for their use.

WHAT NOT TO DO

Kindness is imperative. Do not frighten the animal by being angry
or upset.

All animals must be on a leash or in a transport carrier. Do not add
to the situation by having to chase an animal on the run.

Do not open vehicle doors unless the animal is enclosed in a transport carrier or restrained with a leash.

If you must clean out a transport carrier before continuing the ride,
do so only in the vehicle with all the doors closed. Cats, in particular, will bolt, and are far easier to retrieve from under the seat
than from moving traffic.

HOMEOPATHY FOR CAR SICKNESS
AND MOTION SICKNESS

Status acute: After an initial dose (four pellets), dosing may be
repeated at fifteen-minute intervals for up to four doses or until

condition is relieved. In cases of no relief, consult your veterinarian.

Status chronic: After an initial dose (four pellets), continue with two doses during the trip, if necessary, until symptoms subside. If symptoms do not subside, consult your veterinarian.

Symptoms	Remedy
Nausea from riding in cars/boats: restlessness, yawning, panting, drooling at the outset; loss of bladder/bowel control; escalation to faintness and vomiting; aversion to food and drink; symptoms worse from getting cold	Cocc*
Fear of pending car/boat/plane rides causing loss of bladder/bowel control; prostration and dizziness; drowsiness, dullness, trembling; classic stage fright	Gels†
Dizziness and nausea with fear	Nature's Rescue‡

*Give one or two doses at half-hour intervals before the trip. One or two doses may be repeated if symptoms persist.

†Administer one or two doses at half-hour intervals before trip. One or two doses may be repeated if symptoms persist.

‡Dilute four drops in an ounce of distilled water and give four drops of mixture on tongue or lips. Or hold open bottle under the nose, as you would with smelling salts. Repeat as needed.

CHAPTER 13

Colic

Colic is a medical term for a sometimes serious condition of the stomach or bowels in which feed or fecal material is halted in its passage through the digestive tract. Common symptoms include gas, stomach or abdominal pain, fever, and sometimes loose stools. In more serious cases, an impaction may occur in the stomach itself or in the intestinal tract, usually as the result of the lodging of a foreign object or, in the case of grass-eating animals (such as horses, cows, or rabbits), a ball of hay or other feed, which the animal cannot pass through normal digestive function. All cases of colic are potentially life-threatening; consult with your veterinarian—the sooner, the better.

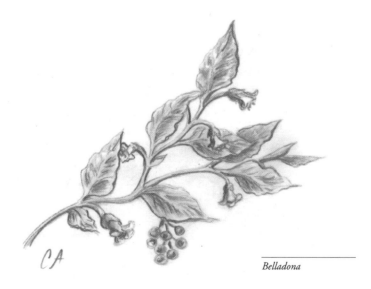

Belladona

A HORSE WITH COLIC

I raced around the side of the barn, kicking up clouds of sawdust as my feet pounded earth hardened by a decade of horse trampling. In the sudden darkness of the interior, I almost stumbled across the threshold. I had heard Nancy calling frantically—just once, high, shrill, with an unmistakable edge of panic in her voice.

I fumbled my way past saddles hung neatly in a row on wide pegs, past bridles and other tack, along a wide corridor and down toward the horse stalls, where I could hear a wild thrashing and banging noise punctuated by snorting and neighing. The noise was unmistakable: I knew that our Thoroughbred, Max, was in the throes of colic. I retraced my footsteps back to the beginning of the corridor and grabbed the homeopathic first-aid kit we keep in the barn for the horses. Kit in hand, I raced forward once again, heart pounding in triple the rhythm of my feet.

He was over at the far side of his stall, sides heaving and head down. My eyes had finally adjusted to the lack of sunlight, and I could see that his face looked anxious and his eyes were staring, with glassy, dilated pupils. Nancy stood beside me, shifting from one foot to the other. "He's been restless all morning," she began. "He bolted his mash and then wouldn't drink any water. When I put the bucket in front of him, he backed away from it as if he were scared."

I slowly opened the door to the stall and sidled in along one wall. Painful experience had taught me never to rush at a colicky horse. Penny, our small white pony, had had colic the year earlier, and when I had climbed into the stall with her, she had kicked out in pain and panic. Lucky for me that I was close by and she hadn't the room to swing her foot in too wide an arc. Lucky, too, that she wasn't as big as Max.

"Max," I said soothingly. "There, boy." I reached him soon enough and, leaning in close to his side, felt along under his belly. His abdomen was swollen, hot, and tender—he winced and writhed at my touch. I could hear a gurgling noise coming from his gut. Something was stuck, and we had little time to act. A spasm of pain suddenly wracked his body, and he began to kick at his underside with his hind leg. I leaped out of the way just in time to prevent being kicked.

Suddenly he arched his back and, eyes wild and bulging, strained to move the impaction blocking his digestive tract. A small bit of thin, green stool gushed out, followed by more straining but no more stool. His head went down, and he dropped to his knees, listing alarmingly to one side.

"Quick! We've got to get him to go over on his other side! If he's going to go down, he's got to go down facing away from the wall. We'll never get his legs under him again, if they're folded against the wall." Together we pushed his head and shoulders toward the wall, hoping that if he lay down, there would be at least two feet of space between his back and the wooden boards on the other side of him. Luck was with us once again. He didn't lie down, but sat up, legs folded under him, in a good position to gain his feet again.

I reached for the kit and retrieved the bottle of Belladonna 30c. With no time to waste, I twisted off the cap and poured directly from the bottle almost a teaspoon's worth under his bottom lip. Under my fingers his mouth felt dry and hot; his whole body was giving off waves of heat, characteristic of a condition calling for Belladonna. And he looked at me unseeing, staring, eyes still glassy and pupils dilated; for him, it was as if I weren't even there.

Usually when horses get colic, the worst thing is for them to go down. It is necessary, in these cases, to get them up onto their feet again and walk-

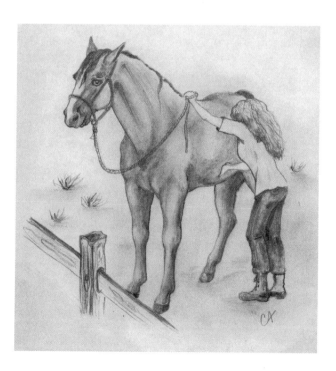

ing as soon as possible. If the intestine is twisted, walking will help straighten out the bowel. If an impaction of hay, baling twine, or something else is stuck in the bowel, walking will stimulate the wavelike peristaltic action of the bowel, helping move the impaction along so that it can eventually be evacuated from the rectum. In Max's case, I felt that the remedy needed time to work. I didn't want to upset him further by rousing him before the medicine began to act; I would give him two minutes. Then we would get him up. Alternately, I watched Max and my watch.

"How do you know to use Belladonna?" Nancy asked while we waited.

"He has classic Belladonna symptoms—eyes staring and glassy with dilated pupils, face anxious and fearful. His abdomen is obviously painful, and the pain was made worse when I touched it. His pain also looked like it came in spasms, especially when he began kicking at his sides. He's also giving off waves of heat, and he had a gushy, thin, green stool with painful straining at the end. When you tried to give him water this morning, he refused to drink; thirstlessness, especially with this kind of body heat is very characteristic of the need for Belladonna.

"Time's up. Let's get him on his feet. If we can," I added, giving one last glance at my watch. Again, we got down beside him, both of us positioned between Max and the wall. "Up!" we coaxed loudly in unison. "Max, get up!" Hands pushing, voices firmly commanding, we worked. He began to rock, swaying from side to side, feet seeking a position under him.

"Watch it!" Nancy cautioned from my side. Max got a foreleg underneath him and was suddenly on his feet. We moved in tandem out of the way, lest he have another spasm of pain and start kicking again. But he didn't. Instead, he swung his huge head around and looked at us quizzically, as if to say, "What are you *doing* back there?"

Nancy led him out of the stall and turned him at the bend in the corridor to exit out into the sawdust-covered barnyard. Here was an overhang that provided cool shade and would be a good place to walk him. I followed, watching Max walking somewhat stiffly, and thought, he's going to need another dose or two before that blockage moves.

For an hour we worked with him, alternately walking him and doing belly lifts. For these, we stood on either side of him, our hands clasped in each other's, and with our forearms gently lifted his abdomen, held it for the count of three, and released. Over and over—lift, hold, count, release, lift, hold, count, release. After the first fifteen minutes, Nancy gave him another dose of Belladonna while I massaged his abdomen and sides in an effort to get the peristaltic action going. Soon he was walking more normally, and his face and eyes no longer looked panic-stricken; his body cooled perceptibly, and his gut no longer gurgled. He still hadn't produced a stool, and while I was confident he was well out of danger, I wanted to give him one last dose of Belladonna; perhaps it would be the dose that finally moved the impaction.

It was. The impaction proved to be an undigested ball of hay, oblong in shape and about four by three inches in size and thickest in the middle. He shuddered somewhat painfully when he passed it, but when he was done he shook his head in relief and whinnied. He began to walk around on his own, doing figure eights around Nancy and me, nuzzling each of us in turn, stopping briefly every few rotations to have a sip of cool water from the trough under the eaves of the overhang. I smiled. It was going to be another of those glorious summer days on the coast of Maine. Maybe later, after the heat of midday had passed, we could go down to the shore to have a swim. All three of us.

FIRST AID FOR COLIC

In small animals, colic is simply defined as stomach cramping that may be the result of teething or gas in the stomach. Sometimes it is accompanied by diarrhea and fretfulness.

In grass-eating animals such as rabbits, guinea pigs, horses, and cows, colic can be the result of a twisted stomach or section of bowel (gastric torsion) or something impacted in the stomach or bowel, usually fodder or hay. If an impaction is suspected, give repeated doses of Belladonna and *seek veterinary attention immediately.*

Note: Stomach pain can be a symptom of having swallowed an object. If this is suspected, give repeated doses of Belladonna and *seek veterinary attention immediately.*

HOMEOPATHY FOR COLIC

Status critical: *Seek veterinary attention immediately.* Give doses of four pellets at five- to ten-minute intervals en route to your veterinarian.

Status acute: After an initial dose (four pellets), treatment may be repeated at fifteen-minute to half-hour intervals for up to four doses or until relief is obtained. If there is no relief, consult your veterinarian.

Status chronic: After an initial dose (four pellets), dosing may be repeated at half hourly to hourly intervals for up to four doses or until condition is relieved. If there is no relief, consult your veterinarian.

SYMPTOMS	REMEDY
Swollen, hot, tender abdomen; restlessness, extreme sensitivity to touch, with pain; spasms of pain with nausea and vomiting; thirstlessness, dread of drinking; thin, green, or impacted stools; anxious-looking face; staring, glassy eyes with dilated pupils	Bell
Distended abdomen, gas; one cheek cold, the other hot; stomach pains with cranky, fretful demeanor; vomiting, yellow tongue; stools: hot, green, watery; sensitivity, irritability, thirst, hot and numb feeling; colicky puppies, kittens	Cham
Agonizing abdominal pain; bending over double; cramps in legs with drawing up of limbs; diarrhea each time after eating, drinking; stools: jelly-like; nausea and vomiting; animal is irritable and easily angered	Coloc
Flatulent distention from gas; bloated abdomen; colic pains, spasms, panting; stools: frequent but unsuccessful attempts; aversion to light, noises; animal is irritable, resents touch	Nux vom

CHAPTER 14

Collapse

Out of nowhere, you suddenly hear Fluffy or Fido meow or bark—a sudden, alarmed call for help. You rush to the rescue only to find your pet lying on his or her side in a state of complete collapse. What to do? Clear thinking and quick action will get you and your animal companion to the best possible assistance, and there is much you can do in terms of first aid.

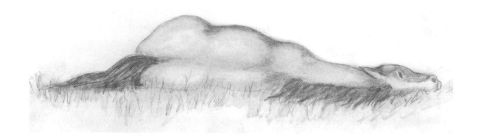

FIRST AID FOR COLLAPSE

Remove the animal to a safe place if possible and necessary. If the animal is bleeding, treat for bleeding first. *Apply direct pressure.*

Firmly press a clean, dry pad or cloth to the wound (if you have
no pad, use your hand).

Keep pressing firmly enough to make bleeding stop. If pad
becomes soaked, put a second pad on top of the first and press
harder. *Do not* remove first pad—this interrupts clotting
action.

Keep pressing until bleeding stops or help is obtained.

Raise bleeding part higher than the heart to slow bleeding.

Treat for shock. Cover the animal to retain body heat. You may use
anything at hand: blankets, rug, a sweater or coat, even newspapers or curtains.

Collapse is a serious medical emergency. *Seek veterinary attention
immediately.*

HOMEOPATHY FOR COLLAPSE

Status always critical: *Seek veterinary attention immediately.* Give doses
of four pellets at five- to ten-minute intervals en route to vet. Crush
pillules in a piece of clean folded paper and place powder between
lip and gum.

SYMPTOMS	REMEDY
Sudden collapse; classic shock remedy; body icy cold, but animal refuses to be covered; faint pulse, weak; extreme restlessness, hysteria; sensitivity to cold, touch	Camph
Classic collapse remedy, lifeless, but head hot and body icy cold; lips, toes: blue and cold; pulse very faint; breathing difficult with panting; collapse from loss of fluids	Carbo veg
Sudden collapse due to loss of blood; weakness, trembling, dizziness, fainting; pulse faint, rapid; body cold, drenched in	Phos

SYMPTOMS	REMEDY
sweat; restless and fidgety; great jumpiness at loud noises	
Any collapse; sudden, with fear	Nature's Rescue*

*Dilute four drops in an ounce of distilled water and give four drops of mixture on tongue or lips. If animal is unconscious, hold an open bottle under the nose, as you would with smelling salts. In any case of collapse, *seek veterinary attention immediately.*

CHAPTER 15

Cuts and Skin Abrasions

Superficial cuts and scrapes are usually minor and can happen anywhere and at any time. Rarely do they become infected or show ongoing symptoms, and usually all that is required for their care is a simple washing and being kept clean until fully healed. Of course, if you're ever in doubt, you will want to consult with your veterinarian, but most minor injuries can safely and effectively be treated at home with common sense and commonly used homeopathic remedies.

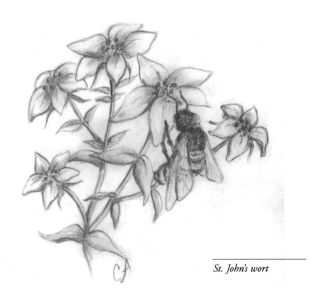

St. John's wort

HIKING WITH THE GIRLS

The three dogs, Missy, Esto, and Peaches, came scampering up the incline not far behind Lorraine and me. We were climbing Camden's Mount Battie on a clear, dry, early autumn day, and as we reached the top, we gazed in wonder at the scene spread out before us as though seeing it for the first time. All around us were the Camden Hills gently rolling toward the sea. Sparkles of sunlight glinted off the bright blue water, and the salt breeze was refreshing after such an arduous hike.

As I sat down on the bare rock to rest my tired legs, Peaches came and sat beside me; I put my arm companionably around her shoulders, and she leaned into my embrace. As she did so, my hand came in contact with something wet and sticky. At once I found the source: a sizable scrape along her side, where the fur had been trimmed away during her recent visit to the groomer's.

I suspected that the scrape had occurred when we passed through a narrow crevice between two large boulders a short time earlier. Missy and Esto were always competing to be first, and Peaches, with her scampering, short poodle legs, was always hurrying so as not to be left behind. The two older

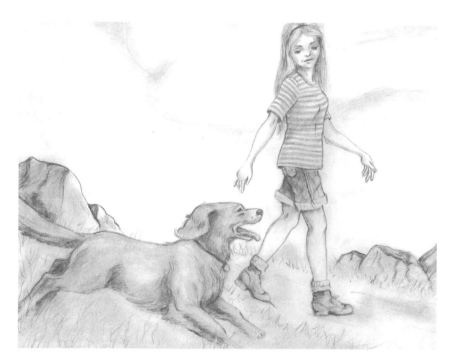

dogs had probably raced ahead of her, and in her haste to catch up, she had likely grazed her side on a sharp granite outcropping.

The scrape wasn't deep, only superficial. It was, however, quite wide and composed of a series of scratches that were slightly bleeding. I washed it with water from my canteen and patted it dry with a clean bandana from my pocket. I was not carrying any homeopathic remedies, but from the bottom of my backpack I pulled out a tube of aloe vera gel and applied it to the wound. Having done a good bit of technical first aid, I forgot all about it until Lorraine called the next morning.

"It's turned red and swollen," she began. "She won't stop scratching it either. Along the edges of each of the tiny scratches there are little crusty pimples. And the scratches themselves are discharging a thin, sticky, and slightly yellow fluid. Every time she scratches it, it discharges more, and the discharges seem to make it itch more."

"I always think of Rhus toxcodendron whenever someone says crusty pimples; thin, yellow discharges; and intense itching all in the same sentence. Why don't you try a dose of 30c right now and give her three more doses spaced out over the course of the day. Give her the last one at bedtime; that will hold her all night. Then you can assess how the remedy is working when she wakes up in the morning."

Lorraine called the next day. "Peaches stopped scratching about fifteen minutes after the first dose. She didn't have the nap I usually see after a first dose of a remedy, but she did rest on the couch most of the day. A couple of hours after the first dose, I found her chewing at the scrape with her teeth, and I gave her another dose. The second dose seemed to last longer than the first, but when it wore off she scratched and chewed more furiously than before. That was after dinner, so I gave her another dose. By bedtime, the itching and scratching hadn't recurred, but I gave her one last dose to hold her through the night."

"And how is she this morning? What does the scrape look like now?" I asked.

"Well, that's why I called. She's not scratching her side or even licking it. She doesn't even seem to notice the scrape at all. All the redness and swelling are totally gone. So are the crusty eruptions and the discharges. Scabs have formed over the scratches, and they look clean, as if they are healing. I'm having a hard time believing that a few doses of diluted poison ivy could heal a wound like this almost overnight. We've used homeopathy for all the dogs for a year now, and we've seen it do some wonderful things. But never this fast. This is quite amazing," she added enthusiastically.

"Isn't it?" I agreed. "Dr. Stephen Tobin [a homeopathic vet in Connecticut] always said to ask the right question, and the right answer will follow. Well, he didn't say it that way exactly, but you understand what I mean. When you were describing the scrape and the symptoms, I asked myself, 'What plant, mineral, or animal product, if taken in a large amount, would produce these symptoms?' And immediately poison ivy came to mind because what you described reminded me of a poison ivy rash: red and swollen with crusty pimples and intense itching with thin, sticky discharges made worse by scratching. Now that you've seen Rhus tox symptoms, you'll probably never forget them. I'll bet that the next time Rhus tox is the remedy, you'll know it immediately!"

"And the next time I go for a walk, I'll be sure to keep on the lookout for poison ivy," said Lorraine. "Peaches' rashlike symptoms are a good reminder not to get too close to that particular plant." At Lorraine's mention of the words "go for a walk" and "Peaches" I heard a short, shrill bark in the background. Clearly, Peaches was all ready to take another hike, and today seemed none too soon.

FIRST AID FOR CUTS
AND SKIN ABRASIONS

If bleeding severely, *apply direct pressure.*
   Firmly press a clean, dry pad or cloth to the wound (if you have
      no pad, use your hand).
   Keep pressing firmly enough to make bleeding stop. If pad
      becomes soaked, put a second pad on top of the first and press
      harder. *Do not* remove first pad—this interrupts clotting action.
   Keep pressing until bleeding stops or help is obtained.
   Raise bleeding part higher than the heart to slow bleeding.
Treat for shock (cover the animal to retain body heat).
Seek veterinary attention immediately.

SEVERE CUTS AND ABRASIONS
   Do not try to clean.
   Do not remove objects embedded in wound.

Treat for bleeding and *do not* remove the pressure pad.
Seek veterinary attention immediately.

MINOR CUTS AND ABRASIONS

Wash out with soap and water or hydrogen peroxide or diluted calendula tincture.

Apply a bandage.

Consult your veterinarian.

HOMEOPATHY
FOR CUTS AND SKIN ABRASIONS

Status critical: *Seek veterinary attention immediately.* Give doses of four pellets at five- to ten-minute intervals en route to your veterinarian.

Status acute: After an initial dose (four pellets), dosing may be repeated at fifteen-minute to half-hour intervals for up to four doses or until condition is relieved. If there is no relief, consult your veterinarian.

Status chronic: After an initial dose (four pellets), continue with two doses or until symptoms subside. If no relief is obtained, consult your veterinarian.

SYMPTOMS	REMEDY
Deep cuts from rusty surfaces; suspected tetanus; punctures, cold to the touch; may become itchy; crusty eruptions at margins	Ledum
Cuts and scrapes; red, swollen, intense itching; crusty eruptions at margins; discharges: thin, sticky, yellow	Rhus tox
Wounds extending to bone surface	Symph

CHAPTER 16

Cystitis (Urinary Tract Problems)

Left unchecked, urinary tract problems can be life threatening. As caretaker for your animal companion, you can be aware of the first indications of this common health issue and act as if your animal's life depends upon it—which it does. Preventing urinary tract problems from occurring in the first place is the best first aid you can give your animal friend.

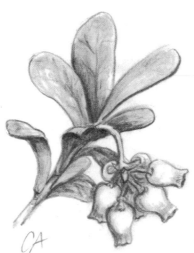

Bearberry

AT THE KITTY B & B WITH THE GANG

Chester was staying at the cat boarding facility where I occasionally worked when the owners needed to get away for a weekend. I had just come in for my first morning of work and was cleaning out the large walk-in enclosure that Chester shared with his brother, Gilroy, when he flung himself down on the main floor and howled in pain.

Shocked, I rushed to his side. He was lying full length on his back, rear legs stretched behind him. I quickly began a cursory exploration with my hands to see where it hurt. His head was okay; all limbs and feet were fine. But when I touched his lower abdomen, he screamed in agony. Gently moving my hands in a downward motion, I soon felt the area of discomfort: his bladder was rock hard and big enough to fill my cupped palm. He was blocked.

Checking the litter box would be pointless; he was sharing a suite with another cat, who undoubtedly had used it since the night before. And for just that reason there was no possible way that anyone else who had been caring for him could have had a clue that this was happening. I rushed to the phone and dialed the nearest vet. Their answering service picked up on the fourth ring. It was six in the morning, and the clinic would not open for another two hours!

I knew of two effective homeopathic remedies for cystitis—Cantharis and Uva ursi. Cantharis is used when urination is accompanied by much straining and the urine is voided in drops, sometimes streaked with blood. Cats needing Cantharis experience a burning sensation when urinating; they often exhibit this subjective symptom by urinating over bathtub or shower drains, where a cool updraft of air eases their discomfort.

Uva ursi is best used when the urethra is literally blocked with urinary calculi—small crystals of abnormal concentrations of mineral salts. The animal simply cannot pass urine, and waste products that are normally voided by the body through urination filter back through the kidneys. Untreated, urinary tract disorders may progress to a state of kidney failure in which a condition known as uremia occurs. This is a serious condition in which excessive amounts of urea and other nitrogen-containing wastes build up in the blood. Symptoms of uremia include nausea, vomiting, and lethargy and culminate in death.

In both cases, an animal requires immediate medical help. But when the urethra is completely blocked and uremia threatens, two hours is too long to wait. If the cat can be treated immediately, he or she will often need a catheter inserted into the bladder via the urethra (the tube-shaped vessel that runs from the urinary tract opening to the bladder) to release the buildup of urine and keep it flowing long enough for the crystals to be flushed out. While male cats are somewhat more prone to cystitis than females, owing to the fact that their urethra is shorter, female cats get cystitis, too. The culprit is diet; a dry food diet makes the urine too concentrated in the urinary tract of males and females alike, causing formation of mineral crystals, leading to blockage of the urethra.

Catheterization is a rather serious medical procedure. It is uncomfortable and likely frightening for most animals. The tube that is inserted is quite small, but often it causes scarring of the delicate tissues. It is not uncommon for animals who have been catheterized to subsequently experience blockage again and again. This may be because the formation of scar tissue further reduces the diameter of the urethra, or it may be due to physical trauma to the fragile structures of the urinary tract organs. In any case, if catheterization can be avoided in the first place, it is obviously the first choice anyone would make for their beloved animal companion.

I had no doubt that in the eyes of his family, Chester was one of those beloved animals. He was being boarded in a famous and posh feline bed and breakfast on the coast of Maine where all things pertained to cats, from the decor and design of the facility to the outside exercise pens, cat-safe cleaning products, and birdsong tapes we often played for their enjoyment. The owner of the facility, a good friend of mine, was nationally famous for her way with cats and was often quoted as saying that the world would be a wonderful place if everyone in it were a cat. That Chester had been left in her care spoke volumes about his value and worth to his human family.

I raced upstairs to the household homeopathic kit that my friend kept in the bathroom. Uva ursi was not there, but Cantharis was. I didn't bother with milk and a saucer; there was no time to loose. Back downstairs, I tumbled four pellets into the cover and tossed them into Chester's mouth. I put him into an empty enclosure with a fresh litter box and placed a small saucer of milk dosed with another four pellets of Cantharis beside him. I hoped that while I went the twelve miles to my house to get my bottle of Uva ursi, he would drink some. Cantharis wasn't the best remedy to use in this situation, but it might help while I was doing my best to get the right one.

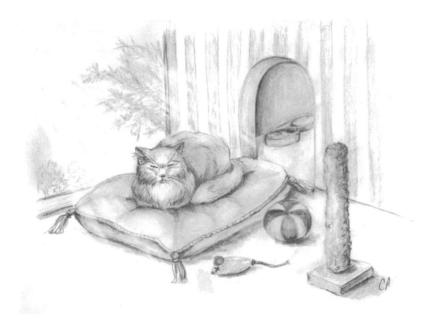

Half an hour later, I was back. The milk was gone, and Chester was lying quietly on the top shelf of the enclosure. He seemed quite lethargic. I got a folding stool and, reaching behind the sisal-covered climbing pole that ran from floor to ceiling, gently got him down and brought him out to the grooming area. He didn't resist. Carrying him, I was able to place my hand under him and could easily feel that his bladder was still rock hard; at this he began to squirm and twist as though it hurt for him to be touched anywhere near his bladder. Over the course of the next fifteen minutes I gave him two doses of Uva ursi 30c, placed his new, still-unused litter box on the floor beside him, and waited.

At the first dose nothing happened. At the second dose he madly scrambled to the litter box, furiously dug a hole and squatted. Nothing. More scratching and squatting, but still nothing. I gave him another dose of Uva and went to turn over the birdsong tape. As the sound of mourning doves and owls filled the air, I heard a frantic scrabbling noise coming from the other room. I rushed to the scene to find Chester squatting and producing a steady stream of dark-colored urine. All the panic and fear rushed out of me as I let out a huge sigh of relief. He was going to be all right!

During the remainder of the day, I alternately cleaned the cattery, fed and watered the other boarders, and tended to Chester. I made sure that he drank eight ounces of electrolyte solution to flush out his urinary tract and gave him three more doses of Uva over the next five hours. I watched or heard him using his litter box numerous times, and each time I scooped out the wet litter so that I could keep track of his urine output. I was relieved at the progress he was making; each wet spot in his litter box was substantially more than a token amount. Still, I kept giving him electrolyte solution with a dropper and doses of Uva, both for their flushing action; I was determined that by morning he would have no crystals left in his urinary tract.

I left late in the day, hours past my customary time for finishing up. Chester was comfortably ensconced in a single enclosure with a fresh litter box and three bowls. One was full of electrolyte solution, another cradled milk containing a dose of Uva, and the third had a serving of Dr. Tobin's specially formulated homemade cat food recipe: a mixture of one cup of meat, two cups of cooked grain, and four tablespoons of grated raw vegetables. I gave him a hug before I left and promised to be back at the crack of dawn.

The next morning, in the gray light of dawn, I unlocked the door of the cattery and turned on the lights. Meows and trills greeted me as I walked toward Chester's enclosure. Several cats, Bee Jay, Kiley, and Moppett among them, jumped down from their high perches and nosed the wire fronts of their suites to smooch a good morning in my direction. I said hello and good morning to each in turn, finally reaching Chester's suite.

The milk was gone, as was half the electrolyte solution; the food bowl had a generous amount missing as well. Chester lay on the top shelf, gazing at me out of clear, calm eyes. Kitty litter was everywhere, and the litter box contained not a few, but many wet spots. With a thud, Chester leaped down from the shelf and raced out to the window that overlooked the busy bird feeders.

I joined him at the window. He sat on the upholstered cat perch, chattering with tail lashing and staring in fascination at chickadees and finches flicking through the feeder offerings to find the choicest seeds for their first meal of the day. I had much work ahead of me on this glorious summer day. But we had time to enjoy the unfolding of it before we began. And for Chester it was the beginning of another day that would be followed by thousands more, thanks to the healing power of homeopathy and a natural diet.

FIRST AID FOR CYSTITIS

INDICATIONS OF POTENTIAL URINARY TRACT PROBLEMS

A history of a dry food diet

Excessive water consumption

> Dogs: increased water consumption from one water bowl per day to more than one

> Cats: any water consumption more than a few laps several times per week. Cats are evolved from desert animals and, as such, when eating a normal, healthy diet for their species, get nearly all of their dietary moisture requirements supplied through their food.

INDICATIONS OF THE BEGINNING OF URINARY TRACT PROBLEMS*

Excessive and increased water consumption, which increases with time

Difficulty emptying the bladder

> Dogs: straining at urination, repeated attempts to urinate without success, urinating in unacceptable places, frequent requests to "go out," small amounts voided frequently, very strong-smelling urine, or any discoloration of the urine from bloody (pink or red) to darker than normal, for example, dark yellow (brown or orange is an indication of poor kidney function). Normal urine is light, pale yellow.

> Cats: straining when urinating; frequent, unsuccessful attempts to urinate; urinating in unacceptable places (cats will often urinate in the bathtub or shower stall over the drain opening, since the cool updraft soothes a burning, inflamed urethra; Cantharis is commonly the remedy in this case); repeated "scratching" in the litter tray without passing urine; small amounts of urine voided frequently, interspersed with failed attempts to pass urine; very strong-smelling urine; or any discoloration of urine from bloody (pink or red) to darker than normal, for example, dark yellow (brown or orange is an indication of poor kidney function). Normal urine is light, pale yellow.

INDICATIONS OF KIDNEY FAILURE

A history of all of the preceding symptoms, which escalate to
    Lack of appetite
    Continued weight loss
    Lethargy (lack of energy, laying around)
    Nausea
    Vomiting
    Collapse, shock and death

PREVENTION AND TREATMENT OF URINARY TRACT PROBLEMS

Feed your animal companion a natural, real-food diet and monitor
    urine output as a part of daily care
    Dogs: Be attentive to frequency of urination, amount of urine
        output, color, and odor.
    Outdoor cats: Be attentive to water consumption since there will
        be no litter tray to monitor.
    Indoor cats: Use a small amount of litter in the litter tray and
        remove wet litter after each foray to the tray. Shake the tray
        evenly to distribute the litter and make the surface smooth;
        paw prints or digging marks in smooth litter without urine
        indicate attempts to urinate without producing any urine.
        Keep all litter trays clean and odor-free; dirty litter trays are
        unappealing to cats and will encourage retention of urine until
        the tray is cleaned.
Have plenty of fresh water available at all times.
In the event that a urinary tract problem seems to be developing
    Change your animal's diet to all-natural, real food.
    Replace drinking water with electrolyte solution to flush out the
        urinary tract and continue to provide electrolyte solution until
        the animal is urinating easily and urine is a normal color.
    Choose from the homeopathic remedies listed and follow instruc-
        tions for their use.
    Monitor urine output (as described earlier).
In the event that a urinary tract problem exists
    Choose from the following list of homeopathic remedies.
    Replace drinking water with electrolyte solution to flush out the
        urinary tract and continue to provide electrolyte solution until

the animal is urinating easily, urine is a normal color, and all
symptoms of urinary tract problems have disappeared.

Monitor urine output.

If a remedy has been given repeatedly over a twelve-hour period
and symptoms have not improved, *seek veterinary attention
immediately.*

WHAT *NOT* TO DO

Do not withhold bathroom privileges. Everybody needs to go when
they need to go.

Do not be upset with "accidents" or urinating in unacceptable places.
Your animal companion is trying to tell you something very
important.

Do not put off consulting your veterinarian. Urinary tract problems
escalate over time. Too late is too late.

---

*Left untreated, urinary tract problems can lead to life-threatening kidney failure.
Kidney failure is imminent when an animal has not passed urine for a period of
twenty-four hours.

HOMEOPATHY FOR CYSTITIS

Status always critical: *Seek veterinary attention immediately.* Give doses
of four pellets at five- to ten-minute intervals en route to your veterinarian.

SYMPTOMS	REMEDY
Urinary tract problems: violent inflammation; intolerable, constant urging to urinate; urinates in drops, much straining, blood; urinates over drain openings, draft of cold air soothes; goes to litter or door again and again; restlessness	Canth
Urinary blockage: no urine produced; bladder, abdomen are greatly distended; animal may collapse; violent pain with howling, crying; unquenchable thirst or thirstlessness	Uva ursi

CHAPTER 17

Diarrhea

At first it occurs occasionally, and you don't pay too much attention. Then, over time, it becomes more frequent, and you begin to wonder if something's wrong. It could be parasites, but maybe not. You decide that a checkup at the vet is inevitable, but she finds nothing and you are left wondering, "What's going on!?"

Most often, recurrent diarrhea is an indication that something's amiss, and we are wise stewards of our animal companions to have it investigated, in order to rule out serious diseases. Simple diarrhea

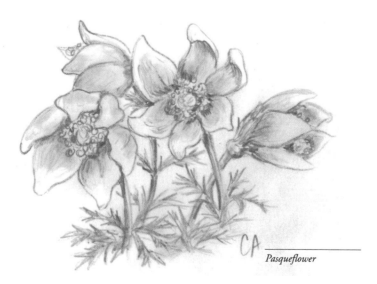

Pasqueflower

that has no organic cause is more often due to water imbalance in the body, and the tissue salt Natrum muriaticum, along with some dietary aids, offers a healthy solution.

ACACIA: THE FIRST NATRUM MURIATICUM OF MANY

Acacia sat hunched in the middle of the living room floor. She twitched her whiskers, flicked her tail, and looked at me through cat eyes that seemed ready to spill over with tears. Since the day before, she had experienced recurring bouts of runny, light-brown diarrhea. Her stools had been copious with a peculiar sweet, rotten odor, sometimes so wet and runny they were spluttery and accompanied by straining. She had stopped eating for the past day and had drunk no water on her own. She seemed listless, lethargic, and warm to the touch. I noted that the water in her body seemed to be in all the wrong places: her eyes, nose, and stools were too wet, yet her skin was very dry and her breath came and went through her mouth with a papery sound. I pulled up a fold of skin from her upper shoulder and watched to see if it would spring back into place. It didn't, a sure sign that she was dehydrated and that her skin was losing its natural elasticity.

I drew her into my lap for comfort and reassurance and took a moment to think. That the water balance in her body was not normal was suggestive of the need for Nat mur. But what potency? There was not much resistance as I lifted her small gray paw with my finger; her vital force, her energy level, seemed very low to me. I decided to match the remedy potency, or strength, to the strength of her vital force; 30c might be appropriate. She looked up at me with wet eyes, not actually with tears, but she seemed worried, anxious, almost ready to cry. I felt at once an urgency to act and a sad tugging at my heart.

I reached for the dropper and the vial of Nat mur 30c, placed four pillules into the open shaft, and replaced the bulb. After drawing up about half a dropper full of distilled water, I placed my finger over the end and gently shook the dropper back and forth until all the pillules were dissolved. She did not want to open her mouth, exemplifying an emotional state typical for an animal in need of Nat mur: difficult and resistant. A quick flourish of my hand inserted the end of the dropper into the corner of her mouth, and four to six drops found their appointed destination. The remedy would

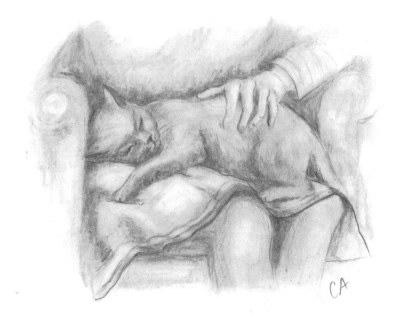

cross the mucous membrane of her mouth and be transferred into her blood system in a few moments. I held her while I waited.

She nestled close, seeming to snuggle into my sweater for warmth. In this, too, she exhibited the chilliness typical of a need for Nat mur. Within a few minutes she was fast asleep in my lap, her tiny cat body sinking deeper and deeper into a restful healing state. I watched her as she slept, this small cat who had won my heart two winters ago when she had shown up in the compost pile behind our farmhouse.

Two years had been a long time. We had played together and slept curled up on the window seat on long, lazy rainy afternoons. Watching nature films was our favorite evening pastime, especially those featuring songbirds; occasionally we would watch a wildlife program that portrayed the big cats of the African plains, but these provoked a nonchalant response, suggestive of bored familiarity. I watched her sleep, thinking of all these things, and as I moved my legs to ease a cramp, she stirred awake.

The expression on her face as she looked up at me was quite remarkable. Gone were the wet, teary eyes, the anxious furrow of her brow. Instead, she looked her old self, sweet, calm, and lively. It had been a good fifteen minutes since I had given her the dose of Nat mur, and I felt confident that if I gave her some electrolyte solution to begin rehydrating her, the crude salt in it would not act as an antidote to the homeopathic dilution of sodium chloride that is called Natrum muriaticum.

Using a clean dropper, I got her to drink about a quarter of a cup of electrolyte solution. Since she weighed roughly eight pounds, I would need to get between one half and three quarters of a measuring cup into her over the next twelve hours or so. We had plenty of time; I was not going anywhere, and neither was she. After she had had her electrolytes, she fell asleep again, this time on the sofa.

Half an hour later I looked in on her. She was having a wash—legs first, then belly, up around the chest, shoulders, and finally the cheeks and face. Finished, she got down and headed for the litter box. I anxiously awaited the results. When she had finished and left the room, I went to investigate. Her stools were more formed and had very little odor. We were on our way!

Over the next twelve hours, she had more electrolyte solution and even ate a bit of yogurt—to replenish the natural flora of her intestinal tract—she had also nibbled at a few grains of boiled rice. I wasn't too worried about her lack of appetite; I knew that her intestinal tract would benefit from a rest, and as the Nat mur worked over the next twelve hours, her appetite would return to normal when her body was more and more able to digest food. I did give her another dose of Nat mur, when she had another loose stool late that evening. In the morning, after a restful night, she asked for breakfast, and throughout the day there were no more signs of diarrhea. Finally, in the early evening of the second day, she passed a very normal stool.

Later we nestled together on the sofa intently watching meadowlarks and nightingales flicker across the television screen. I felt grateful for the heroic healing that two doses of Nat mur had facilitated. We were both enraptured by the visual display and trilling sound of birdcall, but for Acacia it was too much. Her whole body aquiver, she leaped off the sofa, flung herself at the catnip mouse in the middle of the living room floor, and ravaged it in glorious feline ferocity. I laughed with joy that life was good again, all things on earth and in heaven in their proper place.

FIRST AID FOR DIARRHEA

As long as diarrhea recurs, give ample amounts of clear liquids (see section on electrolyte solution for amounts and recipe), but rest the digestive tract by fasting from foods for the remainder of the day. Then, when diarrhea has not recurred for twenty-four hours, introduce light foods into the diet, such as dry toast, meat broth, boiled rice, or prepared baby cereal.

If diarrhea returns, omit light foods, give only clear fluids or electrolyte solution, and wait for cessation of diarrhea for twenty-four hours before introducing light foods again. Persistent diarrhea may require veterinary attention. Once an animal is doing well on a light diet with no return of diarrhea, gradually add small amounts of the usual foods to the light diet until the animal has returned to the food you usually feed it.

To tell whether an animal is dehydrated, use the "skin test." Dehydrated animals will have skin that has lost its elasticity and appears looser, or baggier, than normal. Skin containing sufficient moisture will quickly snap or spring back when pulled away from the body. Pull the skin out and away from muscle tissue. If it does not spring back quickly, or if it moves back toward the muscle tissue very slowly, your animal may be dehydrated or becoming dehydrated. Try the test on your own skin as a comparison. Refer to the recipe section for electrolyte solution and give standard amounts.

HOMEOPATHY FOR DIARRHEA

Status critical: *Seek veterinary attention immediately.* Give doses of four pellets at five- to ten-minute intervals en route to your veterinarian. Diarrhea with copious amounts of bright red blood is a sign of critical status.

Status acute: After an initial dose (four pellets), treatment may be repeated at one- to two-hour intervals for up to four doses or until relief is noted. If there is no relief, consult your veterinarian.

Status chronic: After an initial dose (four pellets), continue with two doses or until symptoms subside. If no relief is obtained, consult your veterinarian.

SYMPTOM	REMEDY
Diarrhea from spoiled food or drink; stools: small, dark, watery, bloody, frequent, foul-smelling; animal is faint, cold, panting; simultaneous vomiting of watery fluid; restless, anxious, agitated state	Ars (follow with electrolyte solution*)

Diarrhea with stomach pains; stools: hot, green, slimy, sour smelling; animal is cranky, refuses comforting	Cham (follow with electrolyte solution)
Rumbling, watery stools; may have mucus and/ or blood with two to three normal stools daily; no two stools alike; chilliness, thirstlessness; mild, gentle disposition	Puls
Diarrhea from emotional trauma (fear, accident); stools: brown, soft, foul-smelling; feverish, chilly, wants to be held or covered; dehydration from diarrhea and frequent urination; skin: itchy, twitchy; raised ridge of fur along spine; animal is fussy, cannot be comforted; thirstlessness	Nat mur (follow with electrolyte solution)

*See Appendix for recipe.

CHAPTER 18
Ear Conditions

They're as prevalent as whiskers. Every animal has ears, whether mammals, reptiles, birds, or amphibians. Some stand up, some flop over, and others are hidden from view. They're all indispensable and a sensitive and vital part of what makes our animal companions connected to their world and ours. All are functional, and many are cute.

When things are right with them, we hardly give them a second thought. But when things go wrong, we may not know it until itching or acute sensitivity alerts us. Homeopathy can be a great help with ear conditions. And sometimes knowing what not to do can be a great help as well.

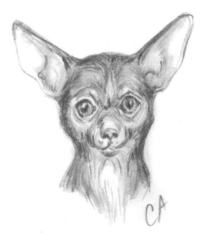

MICK AND HEPAR SULPH

I was awakened in the night by Mick. He jumped up on the bed beside me and pawed at me with his front foot, whining. Instantly awake, I sat up and turned on the light. "What's the matter, boy?" I asked in concern. He tilted his soft cocker spaniel head to one side and just looked at me. He looked all right. He wasn't hot to my touch, and the rest of him seemed fine, too. I got up and explored the house to check things out. All quiet, and everything as it should be. I went back to bed and invited him to come along. We fell asleep and dreamed our separate dreams.

In the morning, we were having our daily walk together in the big field out behind the barn. Mick suddenly ran toward a bush and flushed a wren. That Mick! Always in a rush to greet everyone, big or small, animal or human. I called him back to me, but he just stood there looking at the bush, as though not hearing me. I called again, louder, and he came on the fly. When he reached me, he sat down and began to furiously dig at his right ear with his hind foot. He scratched and rubbed, sending bits of fur flying, whimpering and whining. It was the same whimper I had heard the night before.

Upon examination, I found that his outer ear was hot, red, and dry. The earflap looked dirty; it was spotted with a brownish-black waxy substance that gave off a foul odor. He didn't want me to touch it. My exploration caused him to scratch even more. These symptoms made me think of Sulphur. I lifted his earflap and looked inside.

The inner ear canal seemed swollen, and there was a collection of dark discharge in the opening. The odor was stronger with the earflap turned up, and small pimples dotted the opening into the ear canal. As I moved his ear flap to get a better look, Mick pulled his head away in pain and began digging at the side of his head again. These symptoms suggested that he needed Hepar sulphuris calcarea.

Back in the farm kitchen, I washed my hands and asked Mick to get up in a chair so I could get a better look at his ear. The thick discharge was draining from the ear canal and could be easily seen. I was tempted to wash out his ear with distilled water, but I knew better. Flushing it would only cause the infection to drain back into his ear. I could, however, use a small piece of moistened gauze to wipe out the underside of his earflap, and I could continue to do that, without harm, while the ear drained over the next few days.

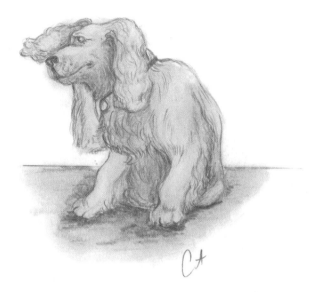

For now, I needed to pick a remedy. It was true that his outer ear showed symptoms best treated with Sulphur. It was also true that his inner ear had symptoms needing Hepar sulph. Both remedies are also used to treat loss of hearing, which Mick had evidenced by his behavior when I had called him earlier. But since the ear was draining a discharge material that smelled sour, Hepar sulph was the best remedy choice for this acute and prominent symptom.

When I got back with the bottle of Hepar sulph 30c, Mick was sitting on the floor worrying at his ear. This time he was rubbing it cautiously, as though it hurt too much for him to touch it. Each time his rear foot brushed the earflap, it would rise up, and I could see that the redness and swelling were increasing the more he rubbed it. I distracted him from his ear by offering four pillules of Hepar sulph, which I had placed in a shallow wooden bowl. He lapped them up, and, carefully avoiding his ear, I gave him a pat on the shoulder and said, "Good boy. Let's go lie down for a while."

Together we rested in the den. I caught up on some reading. Mick slept for two hours at my feet on the cool hearth of the fireplace. I had suspected that he would lie there rather than on the hooked oval rug in the middle of the room; it is typical for animals with symptoms best treated by Sulphur or Hepar sulph to seek cool places to lie down. When he woke, I went to check his ear.

Improvement was marginal. The redness was only half gone, and the ear was still quite swollen and pussy. Still, I did not want to give up on Hepar sulph; I would give him another dose after he had a chance to go out for a "dog chore" and a bit of lunch and a cool drink. Half an hour later, we took up our places again in the den. The second dose of Hepar sulph lulled Mick to sleep, and when he woke almost an hour later his ear looked much better. The redness and swelling were almost gone, and after I wiped the discharge from the outer ear, I could see that there seemed to be less in the ear canal itself. His ear still smelled awful, but the odor was not as strong as it had been. He had stopped scratching and worrying at it.

Over the course of the day, I gave him two more doses of Hepar sulph and noted increasing but still slight improvement. That night I gave him a final dose just before bedtime. Mick sought the cool, wide floorboards next to my bed, as I settled in to sleep. In the morning I woke to find him asleep on the quilt folded at the foot of my bed. He obviously was no longer needing cool places, a very good sign that he was getting better. At breakfast he did not rub or scratch at his ear, and he looked at me when I made my usual morning comments about the day ahead of us. His hearing had improved, too.

When I lifted his earflap to look inside, he did not pull away in discomfort. It was much improved and looked only slightly swollen, with a small bit of brownish material. I washed the bare patch just below the ear, where the discharge had drained during the night. It was sensitive there, and Mick winced. This was evidence of a deep inner ear infection, another indication that Hepar sulph was the correct remedy choice.

In all, Mick had four doses of Hepar sulph each day for the next three days; every day his ear improved. On the fifth day his ear was very much better: the smell, redness, and puffiness were gone, and no more discharge could be seen. The place just below his ear, however, was still sensitive to the touch, so I continued to give him Hepar sulph but cut back the dosage frequency to twice a day. After three days of Hepar sulph 30c twice a day, his ear was no longer sensitive anywhere. He was fine, and I stopped giving him the remedy altogether.

Before lunch the next day, we went out to the field to visit Mick's bird friend. It had been some time since he had seen her, and they had much catching up to do. We stood together looking at the farm country spread out before us. I bent down slightly and said in my customary soft voice,

"Where is she, Mick?" He dashed to the bush in the middle of the field where the wren had her nest and gave a short bark in greeting. As she took wing and flew over his head, Mick looked back at me with a big grin on his face. "She's here," he seemed to be saying. "Right where I left her."

FIRST AID FOR EAR CONDITIONS

INDICATIONS OF EAR PROBLEMS

Scratching or rubbing of the ears or shaking of the head

Unusual ear symptoms

    Odor

    Redness, heat, or swelling

    Discharges of any kind: dark and waxy, watery, or discolored (white, brown, yellow, green, etc.). Discharges that are white, yellow, or green commonly indicate a bacterial or viral infection of the inner ear, especially when accompanied by loss of balance. Antibiotic therapy is a valuable adjunct therapy to homeopathy (the two can be safely and effectively used together), to prevent permanent damage to the delicate structures of the ear.

"Dirty," greasy ears

Difficulty in hearing

Unexplained loss of balance

GENERAL EAR CARE

Routinely examine the outer ear for discharges, wax buildup, odor, and burrs or seeds (remove burrs, seeds).

Healthy ears do not need to be cleaned or groomed. (Some breeds of dogs and cats have very long hair that grows in a tangle around the outer ear. In these cases, regular combing of the hair in a direction away from the outer ear is a good grooming practice; if necessary, ear hairs may be trimmed monthly with blunt scissors.)

If ears need to be cleansed of wax buildup or discharges, clean only the outer ear and earflap.

Wrap clean tissue paper around the index finger, dip into mineral oil (only), and swab out only the outer ear and flap.

Do seek veterinary attention for chronic ear symptoms.

WHAT NOT TO DO

Do not use swabs. Matter can easily be pushed into the inner ear, further impacting material already present and leading to complications. Swabs can also rupture eardrums or damage the delicate structures of the ear. Do not put anything into the ear further than can be seen with the unaided eye.

Do not pour any liquids into the ear.

HOMEOPATHY FOR EAR CONDITIONS

Status critical: *Seek veterinary attention immediately.* Give doses of four pellets at five- to ten-minute intervals en route to your veterinarian.

Status acute: After an initial dose (four pellets), dosing may be repeated at half-hour to hourly intervals for up to four doses or until condition is relieved. If there is no relief, consult your veterinarian.

Status chronic: After an initial dose (four pellets), treatment may be repeated with one or two daily doses or until symptoms subside. In the case of chronic ear infections, antibiotic treatment may be needed to prevent damage to the delicate structures of the inner ear, which may lead to permanent deafness. If no relief is obtained, consult your veterinarian.

SYMPTOMS	REMEDY
OUTER EAR	
Outer ear swollen, red, sore; early stages of ear problems; pockets of clear fluid under the skin; sensitivity—animal winces when touched; animal is listless, fidgety, hard to please, and may whine or cry from pains	Apis
Blood blisters or bleeding from ears; pain, heat, extreme sensitivity; aversion to touch; animal wants to be left alone	Arnica
Outer ear hot, red, dry, itchy; animal must	Sulphur

SYMPTOMS	REMEDY
scratch, which causes more inflammation; hearing painfully acute, followed by deafness; foul odor and dirty appearance	

INNER EAR

First remedy for inner ear infections; sudden symptoms with fever; inner ear swollen, red, hot, painful; animal is restless, fidgety, rubs the ear; loss of balance, falling to the right	Aconite
Outer and inner ear swollen, red, hot; glands swollen; throbbing of pulse in ear; extreme pain, animal resents touch anywhere, animal becomes sensitive to noise, animal is hot, listless, restless, thirstless	Bell
Deep inner ear infections; discharges: pus that is dark, foul-smelling; loss of hearing; pustules in ear canal; craving for sour/strong foods; need for cool places to lie down	Hepar sulph
Inner ear canal inflammation, ulcers, boils; discharges: thick, yellow, bloody, foul-smelling; possible eye/sinus symptoms; symptoms worsening at night, with warmth	Merc
Inner and outer ear swelling; discharges: bloody pus; pain causing itching and scratching; ears hot to the touch; restlessness, with constant change of position; loss of balance, circling to the left	Rhus tox

CHAPTER 19

Electrocution

Small animals, especially burrowing species, are prone to chewing on electrical cords. My rabbit, Hervena, gave me one possible clue as to why this might be true. Often in their warrens and burrows, tree roots hang down from the ceilings of their tunnels, which they chew through to clear the way or nibble on as part of a varied diet. My guess is that animals mistake electrical cords for easily nibbled roots.

Tape all electrical cords to the wall with heavy duct tape, high out of reach. Tie them in bundles and suspend them several feet off

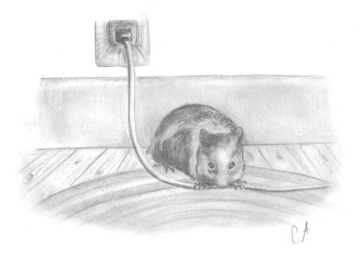

the floor with string fastened to a curtain rod. Don't bother covering them with rugs or taping them to the floor; these tricks won't fool a rodent or a lagomorph. Just keep them out of the way in any way you can.

FIRST AID FOR ELECTROCUTION

Treat for third-degree burns.

Do not move animal unless necessary.

Do not immerse in cold water.

Apply a clean, thick, dry dressing to burned areas—don't wrap, just cover.

Do not remove collar or burned skin.

Treat for shock (cover animal to retain body heat).

Seek veterinary attention immediately.

HOMEOPATHY FOR ELECTROCUTION

Status always critical: *Seek veterinary attention immediately.* Give doses of four pellets at five- to ten-minute intervals en route to your veterinarian.

ACONITE

En route to your veterinarian, crush four pellets in a piece of clean folded paper and place powder between lip and gum. After an initial dose (four pellets), treatment may be repeated at five- to ten-minute intervals until arrival at your veterinary clinic. Compare with Nature's Rescue.

NATURE'S RESCUE

En route to your veterinarian, make a dilution of four drops in an ounce of water and give four drops of this mixture on tongue or lips. If animal is unconscious, hold the open bottle under the nose, as with smelling salts. Dosing may be repeated at five- to ten-minute intervals until arrival at a veterinary clinic.

CHAPTER 20

Eye Conditions

I've seen the worst of eye injuries caused by cat fights. In one case, it was recommended by the attending vet that a cat's eye be removed because the cornea was so badly torn. We decided to give the homeopathic remedy Symphytum 30c a try, forgoing the vet's prescription and recommendation.

What we found most amazing was that the cat would present herself at the end of the kitchen cabinet where the remedies were kept and pester us until we gave her a dose of Symphytum. She continued to do this until her eye was healed. A week after her initial visit, we took the cat, with her eye intact, back to the vet. He said it was an unprecedented healing, likely due to the ointment he had prescribed.

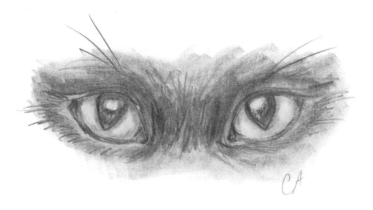

JEB GETS A NEW WARDROBE
AND A NEW OUTLOOK

With a yelp, our dog Jeb came running around the corner of the house to where I was raking leaves by the front porch. He raced up to me, hunched down next to the bottom step, and whined. "Whatever is the matter, Jeb?" I asked with concern. He rubbed at his face with a forepaw and whined again.

I knelt down and examined his face without touching it. Wet tears were streaming from his right eye, and there was a piece of a raspberry cane clinging to the long silky blond fur of his right ear. He'd probably been digging under the raspberry canes again, an activity which I had repeatedly tried to discourage because of the thorns. Removing my gloves, I called him inside to the kitchen, where I could wash my hands before examining his eye.

After drying my hands on a clean towel, I moistened a piece of paper toweling and wiped the dirt from just below his eye. A nasty gash was evident across the entire lid, and his eye was red, inflamed, and squinted shut. I would have to take him to be seen by our vet for a closer examination and a diagnosis of the damage.

In the exam room at the veterinary clinic, Marc looked closely at the gash. "Pretty bad," he said. "I don't hold much hope for this eye. The cornea, which is the clear membrane covering the eye itself, is badly gouged. He might lose it. We can try to save it, but I'd put the odds at less than thirty percent that he'll ever see out of it again. It's your call." I agreed that a pressure bandage would be a good idea, and asked if his clinic had an Elizabethan collar we could borrow for a few days.

At home later that day, Jeb peered balefully at me out of his unbandaged eye. I had no doubt that the pressure bandage holding his injured eye immobile felt somewhat strange to him, but his expression clearly stated that he was less than pleased with his new temporary wardrobe. The smaller end of the Elizabethan collar, which looks something like a plastic lamp shade, was strapped snugly around his neck, the wider end flaring out almost to his nose. It was meant to keep him from being able to scratch at his bandage as well as his eye. Cumbersome and uncomfortable as it was, it was an important part of his recovery process.

"Treat!" I said encouragingly, holding out a dose of Symphytum I had placed in a shallow dish. Jeb raised his head and looked excited. He was an easy patient to administer homeopathic remedies to; the milk sugar–based pillules always delighted his sweet tooth. As I placed the edge of the dish

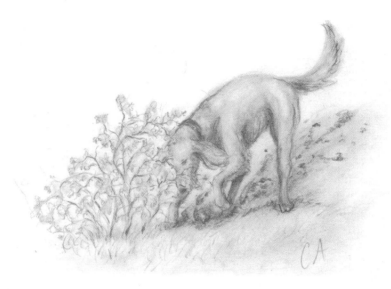

within reach of his mouth, he eagerly licked them up with his tongue. I had no doubt that Symphytum was the correct remedy for the severe injury to his eye; I had seen it perform miraculous cures with many animals who had similar wounds, and many of them had healed in a few days' time.

We went out to the summer porch at the back of the house, where Jeb climbed up on the cushioned porch swing. I sat down beside him and settled in for a rest from the day's excitement. After I had placed a small pillow across my thighs, Jeb moved over closer to put his head in my lap. I put a small folded towel between the plastic collar and his cheek for comfort and told him to lie down. Within moments, we both sighed a deep sigh, and I could feel the tension of the previous few hours begin to slide away.

I had decided to give him Symphytum 30c every two hours or so for the first twelve hours, since his eye symptoms stemmed from an acute traumatic injury. The following day I would give doses quite a bit less frequently, maybe four times over the course of the day, and repeat that dosage frequency again on the third day. We were scheduled for a follow-up examination with our vet three days after the accident with the raspberry briars, and I had great confidence that Marc would be delighted and relieved with the healing that had taken place in the interim.

At the appointed time we were back at the animal clinic. Marc's mood seemed somewhat subdued, as though he fully expected to have to give us both regretful news. Jeb was nosing around the corners of the exam room, completely absorbed in the unseen world of faint impressions that only dogs are privileged to know. Without a word to either of us, Marc knelt down and lifted Jeb to the exam table. He removed the collar from Jeb's neck and pulled away the tape holding the pressure bandage in place. As Jeb's eye was revealed, Marc gasped.

Except for a small streak of dried discharge on the lower lid, the eye looked almost healed. Gone was the redness of the lid; the eye itself and the surrounding tissues were no longer swollen. Jeb blinked his eye for the first time in several days and looked happily up into Marc's face.

"This is quite remarkable," Marc said, as he cleaned the eye area with a sterile pad moistened with saline solution. "I actually had less hope of Jeb's eye recovering than I let on to you initially. This is amazing! I can't tell you how happy I am to see this!" He reached out and gave Jeb an enthusiastic rub on the top of his head.

At the movement of Marc's hand, Jeb butted his head toward Marc's palm and raised his paw to shake hands. "Evidently, his vision in that eye is still intact, too," Marc said with a smile. "I'll just have a look with this small gadget I use for looking into the eye past the cornea and see what I can see."

Marc peered through the lens of a small magnifying instrument that had a light coming out of the shaft and through the lens. "There's still a slight scratch there, but it seems to be healing very rapidly. The cornea isn't clouded at all, which I would normally expect from such a severe gash as this. My guess is that his vision in that eye will be almost, if not totally, what it was originally. You're quite a lucky dog, Jeb," he concluded, shaking Jeb's outstretched paw.

Marc turned to me. "Well, I bet your next order of business is digging up those raspberry brambles yourself, while Jeb looks on from the safety of the summer porch." He waggled his eyebrows at me and smiled. "Yup," I said. "Right after we have one of those doggie biscuits you keep hidden under the counter there."

FIRST AID FOR EYE CONDITIONS

OBJECTS ON THE SURFACE OF THE EYES (DIRT OR LINT)
Wash your hands before examining the eye.

If the object is just on the *surface* of the eye, pull down the lower lid
and remove with the corner of clean tissue or cloth or flush out
with warm water.

Note: A major cause of dirt or foreign objects in or on the eye is allowing dogs to ride in the back of open pickup trucks. For this and other safety reasons, have your dog ride up front with you.

OBJECTS DEEPLY EMBEDDED IN THE EYE

Do not remove the object.

Cover both eyes (to keep them from moving).

Seek veterinary attention immediately.

CHEMICAL BURNS TO THE EYES

Symptoms: Runny, watery eyes and blistering

Test: Smell the animal's face. Does it smell like gasoline or kerosene or other strong odors?

Rinse with *lots* of warm water for fifteen minutes.

Always rinse from the nose to the outer edge of the eye so that chemical does not run into the other eye.

Bandage the eye or eyes.

Seek veterinary attention immediately.

IF AN EYE IS PULLED OR PUSHED OUT OF THE EYE SOCKET

Wet both eye and socket in a sugar-water solution; keep both moist and immobilize the animal.

Treat for shock (cover animal to retain body heat).

Seek veterinary attention immediately. Continue moistening eye and socket en route to your veterinarian.

HOMEOPATHY FOR EYE CONDITIONS

Status critical: *Seek veterinary attention immediately.* Give doses of four pellets at five- to ten-minute intervals en route to your veterinarian.

Status acute: After an initial dose (four pellets), dosing may be repeated at fifteen-minute to half-hour intervals for up to four doses or until condition is relieved. If there is no relief, *seek veterinary attention immediately.*

Status chronic: After an initial dose (four pellets), continue with two doses a day or until symptoms subside. If no relief is obtained, consult your veterinarian.

Symptoms	Remedy
Swollen lids, conjunctiva; inflamed, red, puffy, twitching; discharges: hot, clear, watery, thin, copious; sensitive to touch, light; sties (prevents recurrence)	Apis
Classic conjunctivitis remedy; conjunctiva/lids swollen, red; discharges: pustular, copious, thick; chronic ulcers on lid/cornea; animal is unable to keep eyes steady; worse: light, warm room; better: closing eyes	Argent nit
Violent inflammation of lids, conjunctiva; violent itching; small eruptions on lids or margins; sparkling, fiery, staring look	Canth
Moderate swelling, lids/conjunctiva; watery tears; sneezing	Nat mur
Lids and conjunctiva red, swollen, itchy; discharges: copious, yellow, crusty; hot, scalding tears, opening eyes	Rhus tox
Best remedy for injuries to the eyes—no other remedy equals this one; use after a blow or poke with an object; scratches, cuts on eyeball/cornea; soreness and squinting	Symph
Violent swelling of lids, conjunctiva; hive-like eruptions on lids; itching and stinging driving animal crazy	Urt urens

CHAPTER 21

Fear, Fright, Panic, and Hysteria

A woman once told me that her vet had told her that her cat occasionally exhibited violent aggression as the result of becoming overstimulated by unusual noises. In simpler, layman's terms, the cat had been frightened by an odd noise, a fear that escalated into panic and terminated in aggression meant to ward off any possible threat. It was unfortunate that the woman's face was the only available target within reach of the cat. Fortunately for the cat, her companion is a very compassionate and understanding human being. And very forgiving.

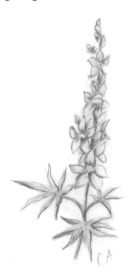

Stanesacre

HERVENA

Hervena scampered into the corner of her oversized rabbit hutch as I put the finishing touch on my daily ritual of cleaning her cage—the flake of fresh hay that went into the farthest corner. Beside it I placed a crisp burdock root, her favorite food. The hutch took up a lot of room, filling the width of the two sunny double windows above it, the hinged top coming to just below the sills. When she was not scampering around, it was a comfortable arrangement for her in the center of our farmhouse, being in visual and hearing range of almost everything that our family did.

I heard a knock on the back door and a cheerful voice announced, "We're here!" We were having company this bright sunny morning; my good friend Karen was expected. I was puzzled, though, by the word "we," since I was only expecting her. Who was the other visitor? I wondered, as I went out to the sunporch to open the back door of the house. I didn't have long to ponder the question.

As soon as the back door was open a few inches, a long black nose appeared in the crack followed by a black-and-tan German shepherd head. It was Rambo, and he was eager to see me. In his enthusiasm, he raced past me into the sunporch, his excitement carrying him further into the kitchen. Hervena! I thought, racing after him. But it was too late.

Even before I gained the kitchen door, loud and decisively dominant barking assailed my ears. This was followed by the heavy warning thump of a rabbit's hind foot striking a solid surface, a loud knock that clearly said, "Danger!" in rabbit language. I rushed in to find Rambo dashing back and forth in front of the hutch and Hervena trying, in vain, to hide her Flemish Giant torso behind the inadequately small flake of hay.

Karen rushed past me and grabbed Rambo's collar, bringing him to a halt. Her familiar touch at once quieted his frenzied bray, but he continued to prance in agitation and began a desperate sort of whining. I did the first thing that came to mind. I yanked down the wide curtain that hung from the double windows over the rabbit hutch and draped it over the top and sides of the cage. Immediately, both animals were blocked from each other's view, and the commotion was reduced to half of its original intensity.

"I don't know what's the matter with him. He never acts like this. He's usually very obedient, and he's never acted so outrageously around any other animal. Certainly not in someone's home. I'm really sorry," Karen added. And she was right. Rambo was a great dog—always obedient, usually very calm and in command of his behavior. He'd always been welcome at my home and had treated my cats with respect and courtesy. But this was probably the first time he'd seen a rabbit in a hutch, and such an inviting and tempting morsel she likely seemed, too.

"I know," I responded. "Rambo is always welcome in my house. He's just acting like any normal dog would. He probably thinks that he's made the discovery of the century, and certainly no less excitement was generated when King Tut's tomb was opened back in the twenties." Rambo strained at Karen's grasp and continued to whine and fret. "I'll be right back," she said, exiting him firmly, yet gently out the kitchen door. Moments later, he was safely tied outside.

When she came back, I had removed the curtain and was assessing Hervena's condition. I had to move the flake of hay to the other side of the hutch in order to look at her face. As I did so, she thumped another loud warning with her powerful hind foot and tried to bury her head in the corner. She exemplified an animal in absolute panic. As I attempted to soothe her by stroking her ears, she became wild and out of control, jumping several inches off the plywood flooring of the hutch and spinning around to bite. I decided that Nature's Rescue would be a good place to begin, but I wondered how I would approach her in her panic state.

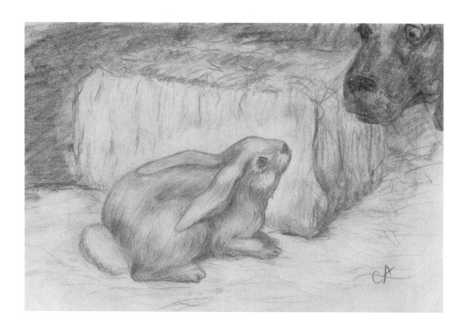

I got my stock bottle from the cabinet and held it open near her face. At this she wheeled around in terror. No good. I next tried squeezing out several drops onto the pine shavings at her feet, hoping that the soothing aroma would waft upward into her nose. It did, and she calmed a bit, breathing hard. I tried again to place the open bottle under her nose, as I would with smelling salts, but again, she reacted violently.

I had another trick up my sleeve, one that anyone familiar with rabbits might smile at: I dropped a couple of drops onto the inside of her right forepaw and waited for her to react as any rabbit would. In typical lagomorph fashion, she rubbed her face with her front paws, dosing herself with Nature's Rescue! In seconds, she calmed perceptibly. But soon she was agitated again. This time, I would have to dig deeper into my homeopathic supplies.

Since she was still in the first stages of fear and hysteria and exhibiting the symptoms of jumpiness—labored breathing and restlessness—and was also resisting my touch, she was a good candidate for Aconite. I rinsed her water bottle and refilled it with distilled water, adding four pillules of Aconite 30c. As I shook the water dispenser to dissolve the pillules, the steel ball in the drinking tube clicked and clacked. At this noise, she reacted violently, giving another warning thump.

I had to hold her momentarily in the crook of my arm, so that I could place the drinking spout in the corner of her mouth. Gently I squeezed the plastic dispenser and a few drops found their way to her tongue. She wriggled in my grasp, and I let her go back to the safety of the corner. After I placed the water bottle back in its rack, I replaced the curtain over the hutch to facilitate a restful environment while the Aconite did its work. Karen and I took our tea to the backyard, where Rambo joined us for our visit.

I checked on her several times during the next hour. Each time I looked, she was resting in the corner; the last time I found her fast asleep on her side, bunny belly bulging upward, long rabbit legs stretched out behind her. This was one of the responses I had been waiting for. I would know that she was fully recovered when she began eating again. Rabbits will adamantly refuse to eat if they are unwell or frightened.

Soon our visitors said their goodbyes, and I went back into the house. As I entered the kitchen and approached the hutch, a wonderful sound reached my ears. It was a sound unlike any other. And of all the sounds I've heard over the course of my life, no other gladdens my heart or brings such a big smile to my face. It was the sound of a bunny crunching on a crisp burdock root.

FIRST AID FOR
FEAR, FRIGHT, PANIC, AND HYSTERIA

Remove the cause.

If it is company, small children, or other animals, escort them
calmly and quickly out of the animal's sight.

Create a safe, calming environment.

Close doors, pull curtains.

Turn off music, televisions, appliances, and so on.

Allow the animal a "cooling off" period of a minimum of 30 minutes before making contact.

Choose from one of the remedies listed. Dilute in milk or water in a
saucer and leave within the animal's reach after the cooling off
period has lapsed. Do not attempt to give remedies by mouth to
highly upset or openly aggressive animals.

In cases where a fear response is anticipated, such as thunder, fire-
works, crowds: provide a safe, quiet place for your animal companion to be in advance of the event. Use the same environment
each time, so that a sense of security and familiarity is fostered,
and be verbally reassuring.

If fear, fright, panic, or aggression seems unwarranted

Look for a physical cause, such as a splinter or needle (it has actually happened!) embedded in the skin.

If no physical cause can be detected by you, a veterinary physical
exam may detect a deeper physical condition. Follow up and
keep looking until you find out what's wrong.

HOMEOPATHY FOR
FEAR, FRIGHT, PANIC, AND HYSTERIA

Status critical: *Seek veterinary attention immediately.* Give doses of four
pellets at five- to ten-minute intervals en route to your veterinarian.

Status acute: After an initial dose (four pellets), treatment may be
repeated at fifteen-minute to half-hour intervals for up to four
doses. If there is no relief, consult your veterinarian.

Status chronic: After an initial dose (four pellets), continue with two doses a day or until symptoms subside. If there is no relief, consult your veterinarian.

Symptoms	Remedy
First stages of fear, panic, terror, hysteria; animal is jumpy, resists touch; labored breathing; thirst, restlessness	Aconite (consider Nature's Rescue*)
Anguish, restlessness, fidgetiness, cold sweats; animal dreads being left alone; fear resulting in exhaustion; unquenchable thirst, animal sips cold water; worse at night	Ars (consider Nature's Rescue)
Excitement or fear causing illness; classic stage fright; hysteria causes animal to "freeze up"; exhaustion, listlessness, limpness; dizziness, drowsiness, dullness, trembling	Gels
Fear or hysteria from thunderstorms, loud noises; animal jumps at noises, movement; restlessness, fidgetiness, weakness; animal cannot bear to be left alone; worse: touch, evening, weather changes	Phos
Nervousness, irritability after a bad fright; deep sense of "having been wronged"; animal is peevish, difficult, unresponsive, wants to be alone	Staph
Absolute panic, fear, or terror; first moments of an emergency; wild, out-of-control behavior	Nature's Rescue

*Make a dilution of four drops in an ounce of water and give four drops of this mixture on tongue or lips. Or hold open bottle under the nose, as with smelling salts. Repeat as needed.

CHAPTER 22
Fever

Not a specific disease in and of itself, fever is simply a condition in which the temperature of the body is abnormally high. Fever is the body's response to products of tissue injury, such as pathogens, foreign objects, or traumatic physical injury, and as such it is a vital part of the body's self-healing mechanism. Low fevers are rarely harmful, and there is seldom reason to reduce them.

Fevers of 107 degrees or higher are a matter of concern and are caused by true physical emergency situations (heatstroke, postoperative hyperthermia, eclampsia, tetany, or Lyme disease). High fevers require first aid. Chronic fevers should be investigated by your veterinarian in an attempt to identify and resolve the underlying cause.

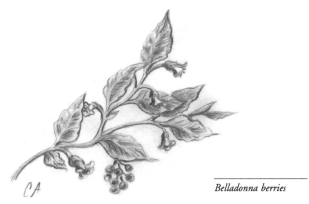

Belladonna berries

A BELLADONNA FEVER

I pulled back the quilt on the bed and arranged the pillows in my favorite position, sitting up in bed to read. Tomorrow was my first day off from my new job, and although I was very tired from working a full week at an unaccustomed activity, I was looking forward to reading until I felt sleepy. I was also looking forward to sleeping in; allowing my body to rest as long as it needed would be like a healing vacation. Before climbing in, I sneaked toward the catlike lump under the covers at the foot of the bed.

"Gotcha!" I squealed, reaching out to tickle the mound. It gave way under my wriggling fingers. "Jane?" I queried. It wasn't her. I pulled a sweatshirt out from under the covers and wondered where she was. She always slept with me, often meeting me as I reached the bed, sometimes waiting playfully under the covers.

I searched the room, then the rest of the house. Where could she be? I went back into the bedroom and called, hoping the invitation would bring her from her hiding place. Waiting, I heard a soft meow coming from under the bed. On hands and knees, I spied her, luminous green eyes staring out at me from the darkness between the legs of the frame. "Jane?" I asked, a slight tinge of alarm in my voice. This was unusual behavior, and it unsettled me.

As I pulled her out, I could feel her trembling in my hands. What was wrong? She came unwillingly and squirmed as I held her. She felt hot and dry to my touch, and she was shivering. She hadn't been like this an hour earlier, when I was sitting with her watching a movie before bedtime. This was quite sudden. As I held her, her body seemed to cool in my arms, and, perplexed, I placed her on the bed and climbed up with her.

As I stroked her head and asked what was wrong, she had a fresh round of shivering and her head suddenly became hot under my hands. This was very odd, I thought. First hot, then cold, and shivering each time I touched her, as though she were chilly. It seemed that she had a fever, but it wasn't a consistent heat; instead, it was more like heat *alternating* with coldness accompanied by chills. Aconite came immediately to mind.

I mixed four pillules of Aconite 30c in a glass of distilled water and gave her a few drops with a plastic eyedropper, then settled in with her. She lay beside me restlessly dozing as I read. Within minutes she began to toss about, shifting from one side to another, seemingly unable to find a comfortable position. I reached for the water glass beside my bed and got

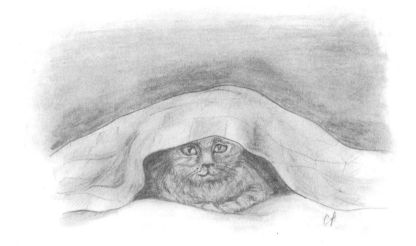

another dropperful of Aconite.

The second dose calmed her perceptibly and lessened her body heat, but its effects lasted less than twenty minutes. Still, I wasn't worried. I knew that Aconite is used in the beginning stages of a fever and will rarely effect a cure. Often it must be followed by another remedy to complete the resolution of symptoms. But Aconite will reduce the severity of symptoms by about half, and that in itself is a wonderful accomplishment.

Now was the time to do an assessment of her symptoms. Were they worse? Better? Changed or different? I looked into her face. She now had a haunted, anxious expression—eyes staring, glassy, and shiny with pupils dilated. Even before I touched the back of her head in a gesture of comfort, I could feel heat coming off her body in waves. She was totally unmoving, almost statuelike, and she stiffened at my touch as though my gentle caress were painful to her. These were the classic symptoms of the need for Belladonna.

I got a fresh glass of distilled water and tumbled four pillules of Belladonna 30c into it. With a clean plastic eyedropper, I stirred until they were all dissolved. Giving her the half dropper of remedy was difficult; she tossed and thrashed and became almost violent in her refusal to take it. This is typical of a condition calling for Belladonna; animals will resist being touched or spoken to, becoming almost violent in their reactions to outside stimuli. The emotional and psychic state is one of a frightened and distorted interpretation of reality: these animals seem to live in a terrifying world of their own, experiencing normal activities and events as waking nightmares.

I would have to be sneaky and quick. I held the dropper above her head and squeezed the bulb. Two drops landed in her right eye, an easily accessible route through the mucous membrane of her eye to her bloodstream. She blinked but did not rub her eye, maintaining her statuelike Belladonna posture. I sat with her and waited, speaking softly and reassuringly. Her only response was to stare at me out of glittering green eyes that followed my every movement. Her pupils were huge, and in the depths of her eyes I could see an eerie luminous reflection that reminded me of cat's eyes I'd once seen depicted in a horror movie.

In about fifteen minutes her eyes assumed a more normal appearance: the pupils became smaller, and they lost their luminous glow. The anxious look that she had exhibited a short while before was replaced with a softening about her cheeks and forehead. Her body seemed more relaxed, losing its rigidity, and she placed her head on her paws and slept. As she rested, I reached out and felt her back. She was cooler to my touch.

I had chosen the correct remedy and was greatly relieved. That Jane showed symptoms indicative of Aconite first was not surprising to me, nor was I surprised that Belladonna was indicated next; Belladonna frequently follows Aconite in cases of fever. The trick of placing a drop of remedy on any available mucous membrane was taught to me by a homeopathic educator at the first homeopathic workshop I had ever attended. It was a gem that had served me well over the years and one that I have never forgotten.

Over the next two hours Jane awoke twice, each time with a mild return of her symptoms. It was her eye symptoms that recurred first, which indicated to me that another dose of Belladonna should be administered. I simply took doses from the water glass I had first made up; half a glass of water with four pillules diluted into it will provide many doses, each four drops of that dilution being a dose. As tired as I was, I was glad not to have to get up again and again to mix a new solution. I was also happy not to have to rouse Jane's healing rest with my jostling and rustling.

By midnight, as I finally finished my book, she was fast asleep beside me. Her body was cool to the touch, and she slept in her usual fashion on her side, chin resting on her chest with one foreleg draped over her face. It was a welcome sight. I watched her as she slept, whisker-twitching dreams crossing her face like clouds caressing a full moon. I felt confident that her fever had passed and that she would spend the remainder of the night sleeping. And that's exactly what I myself planned to do. Yawning, I turned off the light and sought my own dreams.

FIRST AID FOR FEVER

LOW FEVERS, UNDER 105 DEGREES: NOT AN EMERGENCY

Causes

Infections, physical trauma, overexertion

Treatment

Choose a homeopathic remedy from the list given and administer according to instructions.

Chronic fevers or fevers that do not respond to a well-indicated homeopathic remedy should be investigated by your veterinarian.

Give electrolyte solution to prevent dehydration (see recipe section).

HIGH FEVERS, ABOVE 106 DEGREES: AN EMERGENCY SITUATION REQUIRING IMMEDIATE FIRST AID

Seek veterinary attention immediately.

Causes

Heatstroke (environmental hyperthermia)

Condition occurs when environmental temperature and humidity is high and ventillation is inadequate during hot weather, for example, being enclosed in a vehicle on a hot day.

Symptoms in order of occurrence: rapid panting, salivation, anxiety, cyanosis (inability of blood to carry oxygen to the tissues, resulting in blue or purple discolorations of the skin), weakness, prostration, damage to the central nervous system resulting in brain damage or death

Postoperative hyperthermia

Condition occurs after surgical procedures.

Symptoms: rapid panting, salivation, anxiety

Eclampsia (fever-related convulsions during the latter part of pregnancy or during labor)

Condition occurs as the result of low blood calcium levels and
sometimes with alterations in blood magnesium levels

Symptoms in order of occurrence: nervousness, panting, whining
or crying, staggering and lack of coordination, elevated body
temperature, spasms and seizures. *Seek veterinary attention
immediately.*

Tetany (postpartum convulsions)

Condition occurs in nursing mothers at the time of peak lactation
(one to three weeks after birth) and is associated with low
blood levels of calcium and phosphorus.

Symptoms in order of occurrence: restlessness, panting, agitation,
ataxia, trembling, muscular tetany, convulsive seizures

Lyme disease (a tick-borne inflammatory disease)

Disease occurs in dogs, rodents, opossums, deer, racoons, and
humans. Exposure is due to tick bites from ticks infested with
the spirochete *Borrelia burgdorferi.*

Symptoms include high fever, lethargy, lack of appetite, and joint
pain and stiffness. The legacy of Lyme disease is chronic arthritis-
like symptoms.

Treatment: Remove the ticks by manual means, being careful not
to leave the head or mouth parts of the tick in the skin (which
may lead to infection). Give the homeopathic remedy Ledum
in 1M potency three times a day for three consecutive days.
Note: Lyme disease is a serious condition. Consult your veterinarian, who may wish to institute antibiotic therapy. In cases
where Lyme disease has occurred in the past and been treated
with antibiotic therapy, it is wise to give the course of Ledum
1M postsymptomatically, to ward off chronic joint pain and
stiffness that may linger.

**TREATMENT (EMERGENCY PROCEDURES TO PREVENT IRREPARA-
BLE BRAIN DAMAGE)**

Sponge the body with cool water or immerse in a tub of ice water;
ice packs may be applied to the head.

Choose a remedy from the list given and administer according to
instructions.

Give electrolyte solution to prevent dehydration (see recipe section). *Seek veterinary attention immediately.*

TAKING AN ANIMAL'S TEMPERATURE

What *not* to do

Use glass rectal thermometers to take an animal's temperature unless you are trained to do so. Glass thermometers can break in the rectum, causing serious injury.

What to do

Consult your veterinarian if you suspect a high fever in your animal. Use plastic temperature strips applied to the hairless inner thigh to assess body temperature.

HOMEOPATHY FOR FEVER

Status critical: For fevers over 105 degrees, *seek veterinary attention immediately.* Give doses of four pellets at five- to ten-minute intervals en route to your veterinarian.

Status acute: After an initial dose (four pellets), dosing may be repeated at fifteen-minute to half-hour intervals for up to four doses or until fever is relieved. If fever does not subside, consult your veterinarian.

Status chronic: After an initial dose (four pellets), continue with two doses a day or until symptoms subside. If there is no relief, consult your veterinarian.

SYMPTOMS	REMEDY
First remedy to give; beginning stages of fever; sudden onset, dry heat, red face; coldness and heat alternate; chills; animal is chilly if uncovered or touched; animal is always thirsty and restless	Aconite (may be followed with another remedy from list)
Violent heat of the body—heat comes off in waves; anxious look; eyes staring, glassy;	Bell

SYMPTOMS	REMEDY
pupils dilated; animal is always thirstless	
Long duration, exhausting fever with sweats; recurrent fever with stupor, dizziness, trembling; pulse slow and soft; chilly, shivering; animal wants to be held, shakes; prostration, muscular soreness; animal is always thirstless	Gels

CHAPTER 23

Fleas

The scourge of humans and animals alike, fleas have been with us throughout recorded history and probably before. There's nothing remotely like arriving home from your summer vacation, walking into your sanctuary from the world, and being attacked by a billion fleas. Imagine how your furred animal companion feels! Understanding fleas and conquering them is possible, and victory may be achieved by using gentle, nontoxic everyday products.

I've tried it all, from chemical house bombs and flea shampoo to amethyst crystals in the cat's water bowl and tubs of soapy water left under floor lamps. The real solution came from Toni Sanchez, who now lives in Florida with her two cats, where fleas are probably the worst.

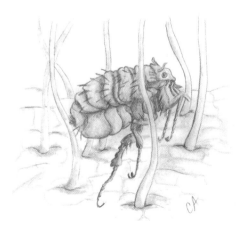

FIRST AID FOR FLEAS

SUGGESTED EQUIPMENT

A good vacuum cleaner with disposable paper bags

Strong peppermint oil soap

Water

Big towels

A large spray bottle

FIRST AID FOR YOUR HOUSE AND YARD

Vacuum daily.

Fleas live in and lay eggs on carpets and furniture and in corners, spending most of their time in the environment and not on your animal (except when indulging in a blood meal). First, vacuum up a tissue paper saturated with undiluted peppermint oil soap (this will suffocate any live fleas that get into the vacuum cleaner bag).

After each vacuuming, dispose of the bag in an outdoor trash can. Use a new vacuum cleaner bag each time.

Spray all surfaces with diluted peppermint oil soap.

In a spray bottle, mix one part strong peppermint oil soap to two parts water. This solution will not harm fabrics, wood, furniture, or other household items. Patios and yards can be sprayed, too. Leave on; let air-dry.

Repeat vacuuming and spraying daily until fleas are gone, usually three days or so.

FIRST AID FOR YOUR ANIMAL COMPANION

Peppermint oil flea bath

Mix one part peppermint oil soap with two parts water. (This mixture is safe for kittens eight weeks old and older. For younger kittens, use more dilute mixture, one part peppermint oil soap to four parts warm water, and repeat bath several times).

Lather animal well with soapy mixture beginning with the neck (so fleas won't travel to the head to escape the soap on the body), working up a foamy lather that penetrates to the skin. Leave on for ten minutes. Try not to get the soap in the eyes or mouth.

Rinse and remove dead fleas with fingers or fine-tooth comb.

Repeat flea bath if live fleas remain.

If heavily infested with fleas

Soak a bath towel in soapy mixture.

Wrap animal in towel (except for face) for ten minutes.

Comb out fleas.

Repeat if necessary.

Rinse with warm water and comb.

Keep animal warm until dry.

Note: Fleas are the source of tapeworms in cats and dogs. Be aware of tapeworm segments that appear in your animal's environment. They will look like pieces of dried rice on furniture and in animal bedding and are shed by the animal's intestinal tract. Symptoms of tapeworm infestation include ravenous appetite without weight gain; a dry, flaky coat; and a protruding nictitating membrane (the third eyelid, commonly seen in cats in the inner corner of the eye). Consult your veterinarian for the treatment of tapeworms.

A note about peppermint and homeopathic remedies: Mints (including catnip!) generally serve as an antidote to most homeopathic remedies. If you are considering a remedy for skin irritation caused by fleas, please be aware that it may not work if you give the remedy just after a peppermint oil soap bath or if your house is heavily sprayed with the diluted peppermint oil soap. Wait a day after the bath before administering a remedy.

HOMEOPATHY FOR FLEAS

Status acute: After an initial dose (four pellets), dosing may be repeated at one- to two-hour intervals for up to four doses or until condition is relieved.

Status chronic: After an initial dose (four pellets), continue with two doses a day or until symptoms subside. If there is no relief, use Natrum muriaticum with occasional doses of Pulex irritans when Nat mur won't work; then resume with Nat mur if and when symptoms return.

Symptoms	Remedy
Chronic flea allergy dermatitis; animal may or may not have fleas; itchy, twitchy skin; small brown scabs; excessive licking/chewing; skin odor of stale corn chips; chilly, alternating thirst/thirstlessness; animal is needy, clinging, and whining	Nat mur
Inflamed skin from fleas and bites; sour and foul skin odor; prickly itching of skin; animal is irritable, impatient, and cross	Pulex*

*See also chapter 24, Hives, and chapter 25, Insect Bites and Stings.

Hives

Hives are simply the tissue response to contact with an irritating substance. An allergic reaction manifests as swollen, itchy skin with or without small, red, bumpy swellings. Homeopathic remedies offer total relief of these bothersome symptoms.

More serious signs of an allergic reaction may include runny eyes and/or nose and difficulty breathing, specifically when an animal comes in contact with an insect or other parasite. Refer to the next chapter, Insect Bites and Stings, if your animal companion shows these more complicated symptoms.

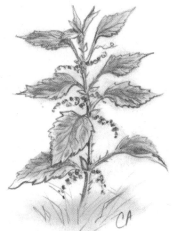

Nettles

FIRST AID FOR HIVES

SIMPLE HELP FOR SIMPLE HIVES

First, clip the hair around any area of hives that has been repeatedly
bitten or chewed, to reduce itchiness and discourage this habit.
Then use any of the following simple topical remedies and follow
with a homeopathic remedy from the list given.

Whole milk
Bathe or dab on with a cotton ball. This remedy may be used as
needed.
Do not rinse off, but allow to air-dry.
Milk will not antidote remedies.
Baking soda and water paste
Mix two tablespoons of baking soda with enough water to make a
paste.
Apply directly to the skin with a gauze pad. This paste may be
used as needed.
Do not bandage, but allow to air-dry.
Calendula ointment (available in health food stores)
Apply topically according to directions. Calendula may be used as
needed.
Commonly used drugs, which may be harmful and do not heal the
root cause
Antihistamines
Corticosteroids (prednisone, prednisolone, cortisone, or hydro-
cortisone)
Ichthammol (a tar-based ointment)
Zinc oxide ointment (commercial diaper rash ointments)
Salicylic acid preparations (made from aspirin)
If possible, try to pinpoint the allergen and remove it from your ani-
mal's environment. Removing, then replacing possible causes one
by one is a simple way to pinpoint the allergen.
Some common hive-producing items
Cat litter
Household laundry, bath, dish, or floor soap; carpet cleaners
(symptoms flare after periods of housecleaning)
Animal shampoos

Animal feeds, especially those containing crab and lobster; also
additives, preservatives, dyes, or contaminants in grains used in
animal feeds

Air fresheners or humidifier/dehumidifier additives

Tobacco smoke

Woodstove smoke

Human skin-care products: deodorant, hand or body lotion, hair
spray, perfume, shampoo or conditioner

Fleas and mites (see chapter 23)

Note: if your animal is diagnosed as having *mange mite,* topically
apply undiluted lavender oil, massaging well into the skin. This
will smother and kill the mite. Apply several times daily until all
symptoms are gone.

Bees, wasps, hornets, and spiders (see chapter 25)

Pollens: weeds, trees, grasses (seasonal symptoms: spring, autumn)

House dust and/or mites (symptoms flare after sweeping and cleaning)

Drug allergies: penicillin, thyroid extracts, vitamins, and antihistamines. *Seek veterinary attention immediately.*

HOMEOPATHY FOR HIVES

Status critical: *Seek veterinary attention immediately.* Give doses of four
pellets at five- to ten-minute intervals en route to your veterinarian. Persistent swelling, heat, and pain or drowsiness may be an
indication of an allergic reaction.

Status acute: After an initial dose (four pellets), treatment may be
repeated at half-hour intervals for up to four doses or until symptoms are relieved. If there is no relief, consult your veterinarian.

Status chronic: After an initial dose (four pellets), continue with two
doses a day or until symptoms subside. If no relief is seen, consult
your veterinarian.

SYMPTOMS	REMEDY
Puffy swellings; red, fluid-filled, shiny surface; itchy, sore, sensitive skin; eyelids may be puffy and itchy	Apis

Symptoms	Remedy
Scaly eruptions—fluid-filled, raw, smarting; acute inflammation of all skin layers; eruptions after excessive sweating; better from cold, but more inflammation; great restlessness; animal rejects everything—food, drink; thirst may be unquenchable	Canth
Itchy skin, small brown scabs; violent itching/licking/chewing—fur stained red; skin odor of stale corn chips; chilly; thirst/thirstlessness alternate; animal is needy, clinging, whining	Nat mur
Small red hives from (or resembling) poison ivy; skin: red, swollen, warm to touch; intense itching: animal can't stop scratching	Rhus tox
Itchy blotches—rashlike, spread over large area; burning heat, swelling of affected areas; violent itching; worse from cold, touch	Urt urens*

*See also chapter 23, Fleas, and chapter 25, Insect Bites and Stings.

CHAPTER 25

Insect Bites and Stings

It's a big world out there. Something as small as a bee or a fire ant may escape our attention, but rarely does it go unnoticed by our animal companions. In fact, not only do our animals have a sense of great curiosity (and often a feeling of superiority) about them, they are also quite surprised when their inquisitiveness gets them into trouble!

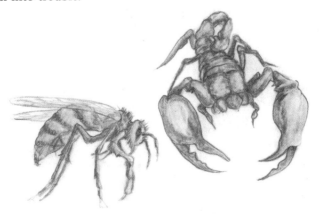

FLYING DRAGONS
AND OTHER WINGED KINGS

Early morning sunlight streamed in through the skylights of the sunporch and illuminated the marbled grain of the gray floor tile and began to warm it. Cosmos followed the patches of warmth as they traveled across the floor. His movements, slow and carefully measured, belied the muscular strength in his legs and jaws. He was an Agamas, also called a flying dragon, a lizard indigenous to Africa, Asia, and Australia, and the membranous crescents on his side expanded like a parasol in the increasing warmth.

We had become fast friends since he had come to live with me five months previously, a "lost piece of airline baggage" that no one had yet claimed. He was a constant source of delight and wonder to me, a creature unlike any other that had shared my life and home. Like all reptiles, he was extremely sensitive to all sounds and movement and he had taught me to walk softly on the balls of my feet so as not to frighten him. Active, social, and sun-loving, I had named him Cosmos for two reasons: daily he followed the sunlight across the tiled floor in rhythm with the heavens, and his body was highlighted with bright splashes of color that reminded me of the cosmos growing in the garden behind the house.

I tapped on a pane of the twin French doors that led from the kitchen to the sunporch to let him know that I was about to enter his room. In a flash, he raced to the bottom of the potted palm tree and quickly gained a higher branch that would bring him to the height of my shoulder. In this way, we began our customary morning ritual of greetings and breakfast—if it happened to be one of his feeding days.

He looked placidly at me out of round pupils and blinked as the rest of him remained unmoving on the branch that supported his four kilograms of muscular body weight. In slow motion, matching my movements with his, I reached out and gently rubbed the small scales that covered the top of his head. His response was immediate: his tongue darted out to my hand to take in the scent particles from my skin. I smiled, not baring my teeth because I didn't want to appear predatory and frighten him, and with my other hand, I held out a calcium-dusted cricket, his favorite breakfast food.

In a twinkling it was gone from my fingers. I watched, fascinated, as the cricket moved under the skin of his throat pouch, wriggling and twitching. Cosmos chewed and swallowed, and the wriggling stopped. He looked at me for more. I gave him one more, just one, and made him wait for another.

In the wild, flying dragons have to hunt for food. Second and third helpings are often eaten on the wing, as it were, and it takes time for these

lizards to catch their meals. I had learned, in the first few days of our cohab-
itation, not to give him all his food at once, and certainly not every day, but
to parcel it out over a few hours. In the beginning, in my haste to feed him,
I had mistakenly related to him as a carnivore and given him a dozen crickets at once. As a result, his digestive tract had revolted, and he went off his
feed for a whole week.

This morning, I decided to try a new tactic. I would release four more
(undusted) crickets in his room and thereby simulate his natural environment. This would also relieve me of what I considered an ethical dilemma:
hand-feeding defenseless insects to another live creature. Each feeding time
I experienced an odd mixture of joy and guilt. As much as I loved Cosmos,
and as much as I delighted in caring for him, it was emotionally difficult
for me to hold the crickets still while he snagged them with his darting
tongue.

As I released them, the crickets fled to various corners of the room.
Some sought refuge in the numerous edible plants that grew out of pots and
tubs from which Cosmos munched when he was not eating crickets. Others
jumped to the low windowsills that lined two sides of the sunporch floor to
ceiling. I suspected that they saw the outdoors through the glass and sought
escape to their natural environment in that direction. One walked back and
forth on the low, wide windowsill, his black body contrasting sharply with
the light-colored wood. Cosmos spied this one first and leaped. His landing was light and graceful, his target instantly claimed. I grimaced in
response, but my reaction was cut short by a furious buzzing sound that
emanated from the corner of the sill. A honeybee! "No, Cosmos!" I
shouted. Too late.

Instinctively, he spun around and went after it, but the coat of the bee
was soft and fuzzy and did not stick to his tongue. Enraged at being
touched, the bee reacted instantly and violently, stinging Cosmos again and
again on shoulder and back. The corner was filled with a wild thrashing
sound punctuated with a droning buzzing sound; all I could do was look
on in shock, wondering why I hadn't seen or heard the bee before the deci-
sive encounter.

When it was over, Cosmos lay drooping on the windowsill, head down
and eyes squinted shut. The body of the bee lay beside him, spent and dying
from having lost its stinger. My heart reached out to both of them; each in
its own way had acted with instinct born of countless millennia of evolution,

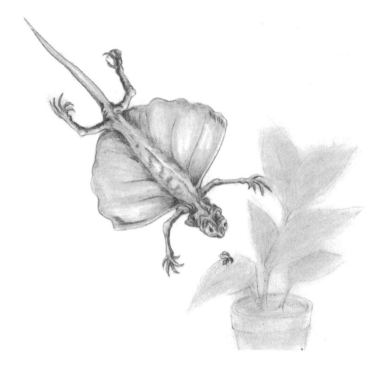

but the final outcome was a no-win situation for both. Within a few minutes, Cosmos' entire right shoulder was swelling, as were two ugly welts on his back. The skin looked puffy, with a rosey-red hue, and he began to act quite drowsy. I went to the kitchen and returned with a dish of cool water and a couple of tablespoons of baking soda in another.

When I returned, there was fluid building up under the skin, and the surface was hard, red, and hot to the touch. Cosmos didn't resist my exploring fingers but winced and contracted his muscles when I rubbed the welts with a paste made from the baking soda and water. I waited and watched for signs of an allergic reaction.

In a few minutes his tongue began to swell, and he was having difficulty breathing, his respiration coming in short puffs. I touched his foreleg, which felt cold, and at this he moved as though he was uncomfortable. These were the classic symptoms ascribed to Apis mellifica, the homeopathic remedy made from the venom of the honeybee. He *was* having an allergic reaction, and with no time to waste I covered him with a towel to keep his body heat in and to prevent shock and raced to get my first-aid kit.

When I returned with Apis 30c and a bottle of distilled water, he was still in the same place, not having moved at all. The bee was silent now, motionless in its demise, wings folded in graceful repose. Cosmos struggled to get down from the windowsill, loosening the towel. Even though the shelf was only four inches from the floor, I had to help him. As I touched him, he shied away from the light pressure of my hands, and the patches of baking soda paste fell off in clumps. That he sought shade, and even light touch caused more pain, confirmed my selection of Apis as the correct remedy: Apis symptoms are worse from heat and slight touch. Yet his body temperature was falling, and I had to figure out a way to warm him without using the towel, the soft surface of which seemed to increase his pain.

I also had to get a dose of remedy into him. I hadn't ever put anything into his mouth and did not know if, in his pain and fear, he would bite. Certainly, I did not want to cause him more discomfort, so I consulted a small book I had bought about the feeding and general husbandry practices of lizards and other reptiles. Sure enough, it provided me with a valuable clue.

The text described how most reptiles lap up water with their tongues, though some, like chameleons, will not; they must have their cages sprayed with water, in order to produce droplets that they lick with their tongues. All reptiles, the text stated, are susceptible to dehydration, especially those living in captivity. Environmental humidity is a key factor in keeping most reptiles hydrated.

An idea suddenly occurred to me. Why not place him in a shallow tub of warm water, to which I could add a dose of Apis, and spoon small amounts over his head, face, and eyes?

The water would insulate his body to keep him from cooling and would not cause the pain associated with touch. And, the remedy might be absorbed through his skin; if not, it was likely to come in contact with the mucous membranes of his eyes, nose, and mouth as I spooned it over him.

I made my preparations using a shallow washbasin, slightly warm distilled water, and a dose of Apis 30c. He went willingly into the basin and sat immobile. For the next fifteen minutes, I spooned the dilution over his head, face, and eyes. When it dripped toward his eyes, he closed his eyelids in reflex; still, I was confident that the remedy would find other membranes through which to pass into his bloodstream.

Soon his head leaned forward, and he took a tentative lap from the water surrounding him. I noticed that his tongue was no longer swollen, his respiration was normal, and his body temperature was holding constant, warmer to my touch. As the minutes passed, he no longer shied away from my probing fingers but leaned into the side of my outstretched hand with each exploration. The puffy swelling of his shoulder seemed to be reduced, and the two fluid-filled welts on his back were shrinking.

I breathed a sigh of relief. He was out of danger and would recover. I decided to let him gauge how long he should remain in the shallow basin and sat back on my heels to watch. Half an hour went by. Crickets chirped in the background. The patches of sunlight continued their celestial march across the floor. Cosmos sat, unmoving, and I sat down, too, relieving the cramps in my legs. And waited.

Suddenly, he moved with the lightning speed so definitive of these creatures. Flying dragons they are called, and rightly so, for he expanded the membranes along his sides and leaped clean out of the shallow basin. Followed by a shimmering halo of water droplets, he snatched a cricket in midair as it jumped from the base of the potted palm toward the window. He landed gracefully on all fours in front of the zebrina plant and devoured the insect whole. I wiped water droplets from my face and arms and, laughing, dabbed at my soaked shirt with the discarded towel. Well, I thought, standing up and gathering my first-aid equipment, he seems to have recovered.

I returned after having changed my shirt, to check on him and to leave a shallow basin of plain distilled water in which, I thought, he might like to play. As I stood up from placing the basin on the floor, I spied him peeking out from under the trailing vines of the zebrina plant. There was a cricket leg sticking out of the corner of his mouth, and he seemed to be smiling.

FIRST AID FOR INSECT BITES AND STINGS

MINOR BITES AND STINGS
Wash with cool water.
Apply baking soda/water paste.

IF THE ANIMAL IS HAVING AN ALLERGIC REACTION,
It may be unconscious

may have a swollen tongue
may have difficulty breathing
may be cold to the touch
Treat for shock (cover the animal to retain body heat).
Seek veterinary attention immediately.

HOMEOPATHY FOR INSECT BITES AND STINGS

Status critical: *Seek veterinary attention immediately.* Give doses of four
    pellets at five- to ten-minute intervals en route to your veterinar-
    ian. Persistent swelling, heat, and pain or drowsiness may be an
    indication of an allergic reaction.

Status acute: After an initial dose (four pellets), treatment may be
    repeated at half-hour intervals for up to four doses or until condi-
    tion is relieved. If there is no relief, consult your veterinarian.

Status chronic: After an initial dose (four pellets), continue with two
    doses a day or until symptoms subside. If no relief is obtained, con-
    sult your veterinarian.

SYMPTOMS	REMEDY
Bee stings or bites like bee stings; swollen, puffy, rosy-red hue; fluid under the skin or hard and red; symptoms worse from heat and slight touch	Apis
Insect bites or stings that itch and burn; site is inflamed with eruptions; better from cold, but more inflamed	Canth
Puncture-like bites, stings; excessive pain; intense itching	Hyper
Edges discolored purple/blue/black; scorpion stings; body cold, especially paws	Lach

Symptoms	Remedy
Puncture-like bites, stings; poisonous spider bites; site is cold; symptoms worse from warmth, scratching	Ledum
Bites, stings with itchy blotches; burning heat from site, with swelling; violent itching; clear, sticky discharges	Urt urens*

*See also chapter 23, Fleas, and chapter 24, Hives.

CHAPTER 26

Mastitis (Inflammation of the Teats)

The condition of inflamed milk glands usually occurs from four days to two weeks after giving birth, is most commonly seen in young females having their first litter (or birth), and typically affects the forward milk glands. Occasionally, mastitis can be caused by trauma, but more commonly it is the result of a bacterial infection, such as streptococcus, staphyloccus, or colon bacillus. Acute mastitis frequently results in the suppression of milk, so supplemental feeding of the young is necessary. Refer to the recipe section concerning kitten and puppy formulas and notes on feeding.

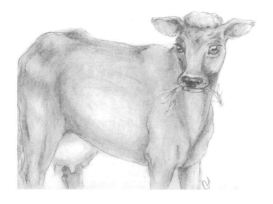

FIRST AID FOR MASTITIS

SYMPTOMS OF MASTITIS IN ORDER OF APPEARANCE

Lack of appetite

Listlessness

Loss of interest in the young; animal may seek a place away from the
young

Low fever, usually 103–105 degrees

Examination of the teats reveals one gland that is hot, swollen, and
tender and that secretes only a small amount of abnormal milk or
a brown or gray discharge that sometimes is blood-streaked

FIRST-AID CARE OF INFLAMED TEATS

Provide a quiet area for the mother to rest undisturbed.

Institute supplementary feedings and arrange a warm nest box for
the young.

Very warm (not too hot) compresses may be applied to the affected
teat.

If the animal is willing, gentle massage may be helpful; Bag Balm or
Arnica montana oil or gel may be soothing.

Choose from the homeopathic remedies listed.

Keep the breast area and nipples clean (with soap and water).

If well-selected remedies fail to act within twelve hours, consult your
veterinarian, who may wish to give antibiotic therapy (usually
penicillin, penicillin derivatives, or tetracycline).

INDICATIONS OF HEALING

Swelling quickly subsides.

Temperature returns to normal.

The appetite returns.

HOMEOPATHY FOR MASTITIS

Status critical: *Seek veterinary attention immediately.* Give doses of four
pellets at five- to ten-minute intervals en route to veterinarian.

Status acute: After an initial dose (four pellets), dosing may be
repeated at half-hour intervals for up to four doses or until relief of

symptoms is noted. If there is no relief, consult your veterinarian.

Status chronic: After an initial dose (four pellets), continue with two doses a day or until symptoms subside. If no relief is obtained, consult your veterinarian.

SYMPTOMS	REMEDY
Mammary glands/teats hard, hot, painful; animal lies still, is reluctant to move, has restless legs; fever, animal seeks cold places to lie; lack of appetite; animal is thirsty for large, cold drinks; general depression	Bry
Inflamed nipples; main symptom of acute pain; stool: diarrhea, green, slimy, sour; spiteful, snappish behavior; animal is very irritable, refuses touch; animal seeks cool places	Cham
Mammary gland infection; nipples itchy, swollen, hot, painful to touch; animal seeks warmth (opposite of Chamomilla)	Hepar sulph
Inflamed mammary glands with ever-changing symptoms; discharges: white/yellow-white, thick, foul, bland; animal is chilly, but seeks open air; animal is typically mild, timid but likes attention; aversion to all food and drink; thirstlessness	Puls*

*See also chapter 6, The Birthing Process, and chapter 27, Orphaned Kittens and Puppies.

CHAPTER 27

Orphaned Kittens and Puppies

If you live in the country or in any rural area where houses and pastures even remotely resemble farms, you are probably familiar with stories like the following one. Spaying and neutering of our animal companions are vital duties we are obligated to perform as humane and loving stewards of the animals in our lives. Millions of unwanted and unplanned kittens and puppies are euthanized every year in this country; they are the true victims of such neglect. Organize a low-cost spaying and neutering clinic in your community with the help of your local animal shelter and a few veterinarians who are willing to provide solutions to this tragic dilemma.

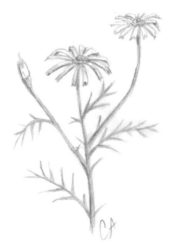

Chamomile

SPRING, FOXES, PIZZA, AND KITTENS

I traveled out of the village on a winding road that ran alongside the high point of the tidal bay and then sharply inland, heading north beside the railroad tracks. Our Sunday Necessity—pizza—had inspired the drive, and I welcomed it, wanting to take in the new change in the world around me. A week before, we had shoveled out of yet another snowstorm, and I was bored with so much whiteness, month after long month. Now, according to the calendar at least, it was spring.

In Maine, the seasonal change from winter to spring is a protracted affair, like a long, difficult labor. And then it arrives, suddenly and all at once, like most newborns. Some say that if you don't watch closely, you'll miss it, both its arrival and its transformation into summer. So as not to miss it, I kept looking for it on the sides of the road and up and down the steep embankment on my left. Sure enough, I saw it. Not once, but twice.

Its first apparition was during a moment of grace when I was driving around the first of many sharp curves. I'm not sure who was working the steering wheel, because I wasn't. Instead, I found myself suddenly looking deep into the eyes of a red fox sitting eye level on the embankment to my left.

He sat there on an abutting shelf of granite, forepaws daintily together in front with his tail wrapped around them from the back. Eyes locked, our heads simultaneously turned together, until we were lost from each other's sight. But in that one brief moment it was as if something wild and still had touched my very soul; I felt as though I had been told a very precious secret. It was one of the oddest and most memorable encounters with a wild animal I've ever had. Years later I still wonder what he was thinking and if he had been as surprised as I had been.

The second apparition of spring I saw a quarter mile later; it was sitting in a narrow band of dirty snow between the shoulder of the road and the railroad tracks. It was a kitten. He sat next to the edge of the road, his fur sodden and stuck to his body, giving him a bedraggled and emaciated look. The topmost part of him looked to be all mouth, for he was stretching his neck as high and as far as it would go, and his little mouth was open in a cavernous wail of desperation.

I had no illusions about parking on the side of the road. I didn't want to run over him, so I stopped in the middle of the road, where I could still see him, and turned on the car's flashing hazard lights before getting out. How many are there? I asked myself, bending over and tucking him into my jacket. He squirmed and continued to howl. I found three more over a small rise in the dirty snow behind him. One by one, I tucked them into my jacket and zippered it closed.

I hurried back to the car, feeling a fresh wind spring up. Still, something nagged at the corner of my mind, and I drove ahead a few hundred yards and parked, leaving the heater running full blast for the kittens now in the back seat and the warning flashers on for oncoming motorists. I searched for fifteen minutes along the side of the road and down in the ditch, listening carefully for the telltale cry of a fifth or even a sixth kitten. Four kittens are a good-sized litter, but more are not unusual; I wanted to be sure. I couldn't bear the thought of missing even one.

Certain that I had them all, I jumped back in the car and headed home. The wailing that filled the car drove all other thoughts from my mind. I forgot about spring. I forgot about the fox. I even forgot about the pizza for the next several hours.

At home I fitted the bottom of a sturdy cardboard box with a large bath towel and placed it in the kitchen next to the woodstove. The fire had burned low, and as I added oak kindling, I went over my mental list of ingredients for orphaned kitten formula. Because of their size, I was fairly certain that the kittens were about three weeks old. That meant that I would have to feed them at two- to three-hour intervals for sixteen consecutive hours out of each day's twenty-four. After the kindling caught, I threw on a chunk of maple and went to make up the formula.

Into a large jar I poured eight ounces of evaporated milk and eight ounces of spring water. Then I separated an egg and added the yolk and stirred until the formula was a light yellow color. Last I stirred into it one tablespoon of corn syrup, which would keep the kittens from having loose stools. I put all, except half a cup, in the refrigerator. The remainder I warmed in a saucepan on the woodstove.

The first feeding with an eyedropper was difficult. Four crying kittens, all clamoring for food, each one wet, shaking, and undernourished. Two of them, the black one and the black-and-white one, were smaller and seemed cold; they moved more slowly than the two gray-striped ones. All of them had experienced a difficult time, but the smaller ones were dazed-looking and acted numb. Aconite immediately came to mind. I interrupted the feeding, mixed four pillules of Aconite 30c into a tablespoon of distilled water, and gave each a few drops with another plastic eyedropper. They sat quietly after a bit, and I fed the two gray-striped ones during the lull.

The two striped kittens ate greedily. One of them had been the sentry at the road, and him, for his diligence and bravery, I fed first. The other soon nudged the eyedropper away from him, but both sucked alternately from the dropper while standing up and greedily drank over five table-spoons of formula each. I patted and rubbed their little tummies, noting with satisfaction the slight bulge. Somehow, there are few things as endear-ing as the soft roundness of a kitten's full tummy.

Soon the other two were clamoring for a feeding, having roused them-selves from the corner they had snoozed in while the Aconite calmed them and brought their body temperature back up to normal. By now the wood-stove was giving off a good amount of heat, and I pulled the cardboard box away from it and closer to the rocking chair. These kittens, too, drank greedily but not as much, being smaller.

Finished, I did the washing up, like any good cat mom. With a warm, damp washcloth, I bathed ears, noses, and whiskers, and before long I had a box full of purring kittens. I knew from watching mother cats with their kittens that assisting them to empty their bladders and bowels was also part of the queen's duties. This I facilitated by "washing" their hind ends with four new clean, dampened washcloths; this immediately produced a small trickle of urine and a tiny bit of stool from each. Having finally cleaned them up—for the time being—I set about making the best use of the remaining free time I had until the next feeding.

I would soon, maybe this very day, have to begin introducing a bit of solid food into their diets. They were big enough and the formula, as rich and nourishing as it was, would not hold them for long periods of time. That was evident an hour later, when all four began to clamor for more for-mula too soon, I thought, for another feeding.

I called next door and asked my neighbor, Mary, if she had an extra box of baby cereal she could spare from her pantry. It was an hour round trip to the market and back, far too long for the kittens to wait. Mary had her older son walk up to my house and drop off the box. It was a commercial baby rice cereal and would mix nicely into the kitten formula, making a palatable and filling gruel. This would be fine for a few feedings, until I could go back to town for dry kitten food.

Mixing a few teaspoons of cereal into the warmed formula was easy, and I made it thin enough to be dispensed easily from the eyedropper. This feeding I did in the rocking chair with a towel draped across my lap. It was a good thing, too; the kittens were hungry and rather messy eaters. Wiping the gruel from their little chins, I reflected that these kittens probably missed their mother. They had definitely been taken away from her too soon and would need a lot of holding, rocking, and comforting within the next few weeks if they were to be ready to be given to new homes.

While they were sleeping, I put in a call to the local shelter. It was a no-kill shelter, and I felt comfortable talking to the manager about placing them there while they waited for new homes. But the shelter was full; there was a great number of cats and many kittens waiting for adoption.

"There's no room at the inn," the manager said. "Yours is actually the fourth call this week from someone who has found a kindle of kittens abandoned somewhere. I can't understand how people can be so cruel or why they are so irresponsible in the first place. If folks would just have their cats neutered, it would save a lot of trouble not to mention a lot of suffering of the kittens that are dumped off."

I agreed to keep and care for the little family until the shelter had room for them. Hanging up the telephone, I made plans to drive back to the market in town for supplies. I would need to get a box or two of kitten kibbles, more canned milk, and another carton of eggs. I would also pick up a bag of kitty litter; the duties of a cat mother are numerous and never-ending, and I vowed that my little charges would go into the world well prepared to be adopted.

That evening, after another feeding, I began to litter box train the foursome. I knew that soon after a feeding, their natural instinct would be to void, and again I washed their rear ends with another pile of clean washcloths while they stood in the litter box. This time, instead of washing away the waste material, I let it fall into the litter. Each kitten got to see his or her own success, and investigated this new development.

The week that followed was much the same. Feeding, litter box training, and sleep. Between these activities, I bathed and massaged them with warm, damp washcloths, mimicking maternal care. It was important to their psychological and neurological development that they experience touch and physical stimulation.

The warm, damp cloths were much like their absent mother's tongue and would encourage them to begin to bathe themselves. Being held and petted and massaged would ensure that they were used to and derived pleasure from

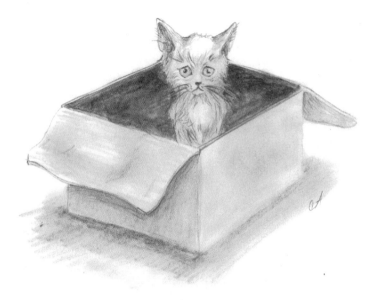

being touched by humans, a necessity if they were to be successfully adopted. The gentle sensation of being touched would also help their nervous systems develop the electrical impulses necessary for them to be fully aware of their physical world. Each feather-light trace of my fingers would train the nerve endings in their skin to send messages to the neurons in their brains, and as their nervous systems developed, they would grow to be quintessential felines, able to interpret the slightest vibratory ripple even from a distance.

I had gathered an interesting array of objects for them to play with. Some of them were meant to develop their response to subtle vibrations in the air around them as well as their hearing. A found feather tied to a short length of string dangled beside their heads and bobbed up and down, helping them recognize ripples in the air around them and stimulating their naturally acute sense of hearing.

I also had made several toys from Ping-Pong balls; these I had painted with stripes or dots intended to help develop their visual field. Cats see very differently from humans. Their visual field is divided into sixteen frames in narrow bands, much like the same picture painted repeatedly on slats of a venetian blind. When cats see movement, they see sixteen objects moving across the repeated bands of vision, one below the other. It is not so much the object that they see as it is the contrast of the multiple objects moving across multiple stationary backgrounds. In painting the small balls with opposing stripes and dots, I was training their visual processes to respond to the contrast of varied patterns moving across a stationary field of nonmovement.

By this time the kittens were about four and a half weeks old, and I had adjusted their feeding schedule to every four hours. They had gained weight; each was about twenty-four ounces, or one and one half pounds. I had also changed their diet at the age of three and a half weeks from baby cereal to dry kitten kibble mashed into their formula, and I had increased the amount at each feeding to roughly sixteen ounces, or about two cups shared among them.

They were starting to eat on their own, making small attempts to lick and lap at a shallow saucer of kitten formula. At first they simply walked in and out of the dish or stumbled over the edge in passing. Sticky with gruel, they would try to wash themselves and one another and, appetites stimulated, would go in search of the source of the smell of food. They were growing fast, and in another week I could reduce their feeding schedule to three times a day.

They were also beginning to understand the purpose and use of the litter box. After each feeding—whether with an eyedropper, from the saucer, or from each other's gooey paws and faces—I would place one kitten in the box, grasp the tiny paws, and help him or her "scratch out a place." The scratching noise would beckon stragglers to the activity, and the others would tumble over to investigate the curiosity. Daily they were learning from me and from each other.

Soon they were six weeks old. They had put on more weight, were bathing themselves regularly, were using their litter box more or less successfully, and were able to eat from the saucer without wearing most of their meals. Through experimentation and investigation they had learned much about the world around them. My work was almost finished, and I had done all I could to see that they were ready. Was I?

Inevitably, I had bonded with them and had many feelings of loss about taking them to the shelter to await their respective adoptions. But all too soon the day came when the shelter manager returned my call to let me know that they had room.

I arrived at the shelter early the next morning, carrying the kittens in a transport carrier. On the way over, the kittens pawed playfully at each other and the wire door of the carrier. They seemed to enjoy the new experience of riding in the car, their first since I had met them. I was surprised and delighted that their temporary home was to be a sunny room that had been built on the side of the building since my last visit to do volunteer work.

A windowed and screened enclosure, twenty by twenty feet, housed nine other kittens, who leaped and chased each other across a carpeted floor or reclined on wide shelves along the side walls. On two higher shelves sat two maternal-looking queens, surveying the activity below. At the yelp of a kitten who had been too roughly swatted by its playmate, one of the mature cats got down from her perch to investigate. With a heavily furred paw she held down the crying kitten and soothingly washed its face, whiskers, and ears while its assailant sought another playmate.

Inside the enclosure, with the double doors firmly latched behind me, I put down the transport carrier and opened the door. The kittens tumbled out, eager to investigate their new surroundings and all the cats that had now come over to meet them. Off they scampered, caught up in a flood of racing feet and wagging tails. Soon they were scattered to the four corners of the room, running, scampering, and playfully batting their new friends with their paws and hind feet.

The other queen got down and sought out the smallest of my litter, the black-and-white one. With a nudge, she pushed her over and held her firmly in place while she began a thorough washing, first of the kitten's eyes, cheeks, and whiskers and then advancing to the more complicated and sensitive ears. She was greeting the new kitten, comforting her and placing her scent with saliva on the kitten's fur. She was claiming it for her own. I knelt down and watched, relief flooding through me. Everything was going to be okay I realized, as I heard the kitten purring.

FIRST AID FOR
ORPHANED KITTENS AND PUPPIES

Appropriate environment
    Supportive environmental temperature
        Birth to fifth day, keep temperature 85–90 degrees Fahrenheit.
        Decrease gradually to 80 degrees Fahrenheit by seventh to
            tenth day.
        Decrease gradually to 75 degrees Fahrenheit by four week of age.
        Keep area free from drafts and provide a warm floor.
    Peace and quiet

Provide an area that is undisturbed by noises, excessive vibrations, and foot traffic.

Nest boxes

House in cardboard carton or transport kennel lined with towels on the bottom and a length of towel rolled and placed
along the sides.

During the first two to three weeks of age, include several rolled-up
washcloths, tied securely with string to provide sleepy young with
quiet nests to rest undisturbed by their more restless or energetic
siblings.

Preparation of formula and feeding

Formula, preparation utensils, and feeding equipment must all be
sanitary (washed with soap and water then thoroughly rinsed).

To prevent spoilage, prepare no more formula than can be used
within a twenty-four hour period.

Bottle in amount required for each feeding.

Refrigerate bottles until needed for use.

Warm formula to near 100 degrees Fahrenheit, or about body
temperature (formula will feel neither warm nor cold to the
touch).

Feed amounts according to ages and appetites using proper feeding techniques.

Follow instructions given in recipe section for kitten and puppy
formula and see notes on feeding at the end of text.

Nutrition

Observation of stool quality and consistency

As puppies and kittens develop over the first four weeks of life,
there is a correlation between steady weight gain and the
increasing firmness of the stool.

If all young are together in a nest box and diarrhea is seen in
the box, you may wish to separate the young in individual
compartments using the cloth bundles to determine which
one has loose stools.

If diarrhea develops, modify infant formula (for those young
only) by reducing the amount of water used in the formula
by one half. When diarrhea ceases, gradually increase the
water content of the formula by one tablespoon per day

until you are feeding the standard recipe for the substitute formula.

Daily activities, exercise, and grooming

During the first week of life, most young rely primarily on instinct to meet their basic needs, yet the caregiver must stimulate these basic instincts.

For the first few days of life, it is necessary to artificially stimulate urination and defecation after each feeding. This may be accomplished by using a clean washcloth dampened in warm water to gently wipe the area (to stimulate voiding) and then to clean away the urine and feces. This technique mimics the work done by the mother with her mouth.

Bathing puppies and kittens with a clean washcloth dampened in warm water, washing their faces and paws, stimulates their sense of touch and encourages their enjoyment of being touched. This is a very important step in preparation for their being adopted. Gentle massage may also be done, using a soft, dry cloth just after they awake and while the formula is being warmed. Such passive exercise stimulates circulation.

A small amount of baby oil worked into the coat will alleviate dry skin.

When newborn puppies and kittens are not eating, they should be sleeping.

HOMEOPATHY FOR
ORPHANED KITTENS AND PUPPIES

Status critical: *Seek veterinary attention immediately.* Give doses of four pellets at five- to ten-minute intervals en route to veterinarian. If in doubt, *seek veterinary attention immediately.*

Status acute: After an initial dose (four pellets), treatment may be repeated at fifteen-minute to half-hour intervals for up to four doses or until relief is obtained. If there is no relief, *seek veterinary attention immediately.*

Status chronic: After an initial dose (four pellets), continue with two doses a day or until symptoms subside. If there is no relief, consult your veterinarian.

Symptoms	Remedy
Difficult birth process; newborn is cold and slow to start moving	Aconite (consider Nature's Rescue)
Slow bone growth, anemia, and wasting; flabby, with cold extremities and feeble digestion; great hunger with thirst and gas; loose stools, green and spluttery; animal wants to nurse all the time; animal vomits easily	Calc phos*
Difficult birth process; newborn is cold and slow to start moving; dazed or numb	Nature's Rescue†

*Give remedy daily or every other day; offer nutritional support in the form of calcium-rich foods (yogurt, milk, cheese) and vitamin D (cod-liver oil—one-half to one teaspoon daily). If Calc phos does not help, try Lycopodium, which is not included in this manual's remedy list, for symptoms of malnutrition, emaciation, weakness, and lack of body heat, and hunger satiated after only a mouthful. Other symptoms of Lycopodium resemble those of Calc phos, except Calc phos is *wasting* and Lycopodium is *emaciated.*

†Dilute four drops in distilled water and rub on nose. Or hold open bottle under nose, as with smelling salts. Dose may be repeated a few times at fifteen-minute intervals. If there is no response after 15 minutes, *seek veterinary attention immediately.* See also the Appendix for the recipe for kitten and puppy milk replacement formula.

CHAPTER 28

Pain

A sudden shrill bark, meow, screech, or growl and you're certain something's wrong. But sometimes pain is not accompanied by a verbal indication. Instead, it may manifest as silent withdrawal and disinclination to groom, eat, or partake in activities that usually bring great enjoyment. If you suspect that your animal companion is experiencing pain, consult your veterinarian as soon as possible. En route to the appointment, after diagnosis, and during treatment homeopathic remedies can be very helpful. But in all cases of pain or suspect pain, a diagnosis by a qualified veterinarian is mandatory.

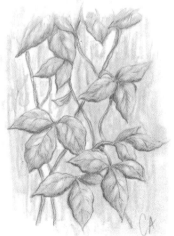

Poison Ivy

145

FIRST AID FOR PAIN

INDICATION(S) OF PAIN

Mental indications

Sudden unwarranted or unusual aggression, especially when touched or approached.

Barking, meowing, biting, scratching, or lashing out

Withdrawal

Lack of engagement in usual activities

Resistance or reluctance to be touched or to interact with others

Hiding in closets, under furniture, or in other remote and dark places

Physical indications

Lack of appetite, refusal to eat, or beginning to eat and then stopping after a few mouthfuls

Sudden lack of interest in grooming

Sudden poor toilet habits or difficulty in voiding

Voiding in unacceptable places

Urgent call to void, increased frequency, or crying out when voiding bladder or bowels

Infrequent emptying of bladder or bowels with intolerance for being touched or lethargy

WHAT TO DO

Remain calm.

Quiet the environment.

Turn off music and televisions; reduce all noise.

Gently place animal in travel carrier for transport to your veterinarian. This will make the animal feel safe.

Wear heavy gloves, if necessary; avoid personal injury.

In extreme situations, Nature's Rescue can be helpful for both animal and handler.

Call your veterinarian.

Explain the situation as clearly as possible and ask for detailed instructions about what to do next.

Follow his/her instructions for immediate transport or for what to do during the wait for the appointment time.

Choose one of the homeopathic remedies from the list given and
   follow instructions for frequency of dosing.

WHAT *NOT* TO DO

Do *not* agitate or upset the animal. Be reassuring; speak in a calm,
   soft voice and maintain a composed manner.

Do *not* ignore pain symptoms. Delay in seeking medical attention
   may put the life of your animal companion at risk.

HOMEOPATHY FOR PAIN

Status critical: *Seek veterinary attention immediately.* Give doses of four
   pellets at five- to ten-minute intervals en route to your veterinarian.

Status acute: After an initial dose (four pellets), dosing may be
   repeated at fifteen-minute intervals for up to four doses or until
   condition is relieved. If there is no response, *seek veterinary attention immediately.*

Status chronic: After an initial dose (four pellets), dosing may be
   repeated at half-hour intervals for up to four doses or until symptoms
   subside. If symptoms do not subside, consult your veterinarian.

SYMPTOMS	REMEDY
Sudden pains—any type, any reason; intolerable and violent—they drive animal crazy; animal is fearful of touch or help; wild tossing about	Aconite (consider Nature's Rescue)
Pain with furious excitement or belligerence; pain with twitching, convulsions; skin hot, red; face flushed, extremely anxious; dry mouth/throat, aversion to water; delirious tossing about from pain	Bell
Severe pain causing doubling up; animal is peevish, spiteful, snappish, restless; animal is easily angered at least touch, motion	Cham

Symptoms	Remedy
Pain in extremities—toes, tail; numbness or spasms; nerve pain from crushing blows; nausea, vomiting, and thirst	Hyper
Pain with stiffness; animal stretches out legs for relief or must move/change position for relief; dizziness on rising; loss of appetite, unquenchable thirst; nightly aggravation, animal will not stay in bed; symptoms worse: morning on rising	Rhus tox
Pain with fear, terror; first moments of emergency; wild, out-of-control behavior	Nature's Rescue*

*Make a dilution of four drops in an ounce of water and give four drops of this mixture on tongue or lips. Or hold open bottle under the nose, as with smelling salts. Repeat as needed.

CHAPTER 29

Poisoning

Animal poisoning is one of the most serious medical emergencies that you may ever have to cope with. Immediate contact with a poison control center may avert death, but a veterinarian is your most valuable ally when faced with the possible poisoning of an animal companion. The best way to deal with this type of emergency is to prevent it from ever happening in the first place. Keep all poisons out of reach, in locked cabinets if possible. Reduce your reliance on toxic substances in your home environment; replace poisonous substances with nontoxic alternatives and always know the location of your animal companion and what he or she is doing.

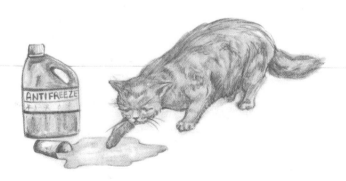

FIRST AID FOR POISONING

CALL ANIMAL POISON CONTROL

Animal Poison Control (Georgia) 1-900-680-0000 ($20 for the first five minutes, $2.95 for each additional minute) or 1-800-548-2423 ($30 flat fee).

Seek veterinary attention immediately.

Animals may eat poisons or drink them out of puddles or even absorb them through the pads of their feet. Here's a partial list and how to figure out which poison your pet has been in contact with.

Kerosene or gasoline: Smell the animal's breath and feet. Look for "rainbow" puddles. Compare the smell of the puddle with the smell of animal's breath.

Antifreeze: This is the *most poisonous* substance to all animals. They like it because it tastes sweet! Their breath or feet will smell sweet. Look for pink, red, or yellow-green puddles.

Batteries or acids: Look for burn marks (blisters) on mouth and feet. Animals walk through it on the ground and get it in their mouths when they wash off their feet.

Also consider **lawn sprays, garden insecticides,** and **car oil.**

WHAT TO DO

If conscious

Turn animal's head to the side, and drain out mouth.

Identify the poison.

Dilute poison with water; make animal drink one half glass of water. *Don't do this if you suspect pet has ingested acids!* Rinse with water only. You don't want the animal to swallow acids.

Treat for shock (cover the animal to retain body heat).

Call Poison Control and follow their instructions.

Seek veterinary attention immediately.

If unconscious

Place animal on its side and let mouth drain.

Check breathing (feel, look, listen)

Treat for shock (cover animal to retain body heat).

Call Poison Control and follow their instructions.

Seek veterinary attention immediately.

IF AN ANIMAL IS HAVING A CONVULSION FROM POISONING
Stay with the animal.
Do not restrain the animal.
Do not put anything in the mouth.
Remove collar.
Call Poison Control and follow their instructions.

HOMEOPATHY FOR POISONING

Status always critical: *Seek veterinary attention immediately.* Give doses of four pellets at five- to ten-minute intervals en route to your veterinarian.

SYMPTOMS	REMEDY
Anxiety, restlessness, and weakness; great fear with cold sweat; coldness of body parts; constriction of air passages, wheezing respiration; simultaneous vomiting and diarrhea—dark, bloody, frothy, and offensive	Ars
Hypersensitivity and irritability; digestive disturbances, convulsions; shallow, oppressed breathing; nausea and vomiting with much retching; scanty diarrhea with much urging; symptoms worse from touch, movement	Nux vom

CHAPTER 30

Punctures

Puncture wounds are commonly the result of an accident that we do not witness firsthand. Usually, after infection has set in, we notice an animal limping or excessively licking a paw—then we investigate. Often we will find a small hole, closed over, swollen, and hot to the touch. Physical removal of splinters and other objects is common sense; soaking in warm water and salt or Epsom salts is also helpful. Puncture wounds are one first-aid situation where homeopathic remedies have an excellent application.

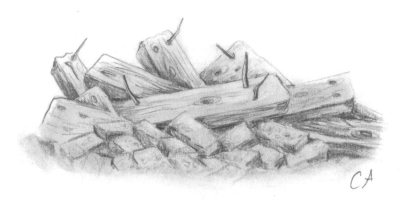

FIRST AID FOR PUNCTURES

SEVERE PUNCTURES
Do not remove embedded objects.
If bleeding is severe, *apply direct pressure.*

Firmly press a clean, dry pad or cloth to the wound (if you have no pad, use your hand).

Keep pressing firmly, enough to make bleeding stop. If pad becomes soaked, put a second pad on top of the first and press harder. *Do not* remove the first pad—this interrupts clotting action.

Keep pressing until bleeding stops or help is obtained.

Raise bleeding part higher than the heart to slow bleeding.

Treat for shock. Cover the animal to retain body heat.
Seek veterinary attention immediately.

MINOR PUNCTURES
Flush out with hydrogen peroxide.
Apply bandage.

HOMEOPATHY FOR PUNCTURES

Status critical: *Seek veterinary attention immediately.* Give doses of four pellets at five- to ten-minute intervals en route to your veterinarian.

Status acute: After an initial dose (four pellets), treatment may be repeated at half hourly to hourly intervals for up to four doses or until relief is obtained. If there is no response, consult your veterinarian.

Status chronic: After an initial dose (four pellets), continue with two doses a day or until symptoms subside. If there is no response, consult your veterinarian.

Symptoms	Remedy
Deep punctures with bruising; infected punctures—pus, low fever; itching, burning with eruptions of small pimples;	Arnica

Symptoms	Remedy
animal is nervous and cannot bear pain; animal wants to be left alone	
A classic puncture remedy, especially for wounds that close up immediately; useful in tetanus; hair falls out from injuries; extremely painful wound; symptoms worse from touch	Hyper
A classic puncture remedy; wounded part is cold; muscles twitch near wound; thick, pustular discharges	Ledum

CHAPTER 31

Seizures or Fits

Seizures can occur for many different reasons. Blows to the head resulting in blood clots in the brain, poisoning, epilepsy, becoming overheated, and brain tumors are just some of the causes. Diagnosis of the underlying cause is a must, and your veterinarian is skilled in finding answers. Once the cause is determined, homeopathic remedies can provide valuable relief to both your animal companion and you in your anxiety when handling this difficult situation.

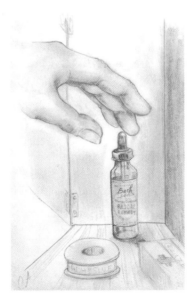

Nature's Rescue

FLOWER ESSENCE TO THE RESCUE

An odd scrabbling sound came from the kitchen into the living room, where I was sitting at my desk writing a long-overdue letter to my friend Jeanette in Newfoundland. Brow wrinkled in puzzlement, I got up to investigate. My cat McTavish was having another seizure and was trying to outrun it by climbing to the top of the kitchen cabinets, where they came within inches of the ceiling. At least that's the impression I always got when he did this. I knew that he was likely only seeking a small, dark place, since small places seem to be comforting to animals experiencing siezures and less light lessens their severity. But every time he did this, my heart would race in panic and fright that he should fall before I could climb up there and get him.

I leaped into action, instituting my routine. He'd done this climbing act so many times that I was now able to outdistance him and arrive at his appointed destination a second before he did. I made a quick grab for the closest kitchen chair while almost simultaneously pushing it toward the counter. One leg up, reaching with outstretched hands so I could catch him if he fell; then the other leg up onto the counter, and finally he stumbled into my waiting hands.

Now came the most difficult part—getting down. Already he was contorted, muscles contracted in what must surely be a painful posture, body twisted forward, his head almost touching his chest, face pulled back in a contracted grimace. I clutched him to my chest and opened a cabinet door with my free hand. I knew better than to think the hinges were very strong, and I'm sure the craftsman who built it never thought it might someday be used as a handhold. But I had reinforced the hinges myself and tried this before, more times than I wanted to; once again, it helped me keep my balance as I gained first the waiting kitchen chair and finally, thankfully, the floor.

I raced with him into my bedroom. Before placing him on the bed, I pulled down the shade to darken the room. As I lay down beside him, I reached for the bottle of diluted Nature's Rescue I kept on the nightstand for just this purpose. With a deft twist the cap and dropper were off and the remedy was ready. Cradling him in my arm, enfolding him with the touch of my body, I lay with him and crooned softly, "It's okay. I'm here. It's going to be okay. I've got you now."

As I held the open bottle under his nose, his breathing slowed, and I watched his face begin to relax. In less than a minute he was no longer con-

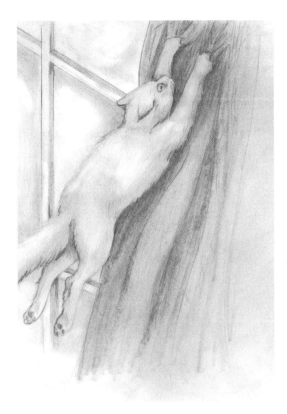

torted. At this juncture, he tried to get up, and from past experience I knew he would try to go into the other room. But it was still too soon for him to be walking around. If he should reenter the bright, sunny kitchen, his seizure might return, with greater intensity, and there was always the risk of his bumping his head on a door casing or baseboard heater if he was still not fully aware of his surroundings. Gently I made him stay on the bed by muddling his efforts to get to his feet—I placed my hands under his thighs and pushed his legs out from under him. "Stay here," I said. "We're almost done." I never knew if he could hear me talking to him during one of these episodes, but it was an emotional reaction borne out of my need to reassure him, and in doing my best I was likewise reassured.

I felt certain that he was conscious enough to take a few drops of Nature's Rescue under his lip without breathing the liquid into his lungs, and I tucked the end of the dropper under his bottom lip and gently squeezed the bulb. At this, he stopped struggling and lay down beside me.

We lay there together for five or six minutes—he staring blankly straight ahead and I taking deep breaths, grateful we had come through another seizure episode with the help of a flower essence.

I remembered the days before I knew about this product; McTavish spent his life enveloped in a barbiturate fog, and the seizures came anyway, despite the daily heavy doses of medication. I had heard that there was a flower essence that could lessen the severity of a seizure and if given early enough—at the beginning of an episode—could cut it short or even reduce the episode by half. I decided to give it a try and was amazed at the results. Since then, there has been a ready-to-use bottle in every quadrant of our house, all within easy reach. My stock bottle, now three years old, was still nearly two-thirds full.

McTavish struggled under my arms, waking me from my reverie. I let him sit up but still cradled him within my arms and looked into his face. He looked very much his usual self and gazed back at me out of yellow eyes and blinked. As always, he seemed puzzled about why we were on the bed, and he wanted to get down, *now.* I let him go, following steathily behind, and watched him walk toward his water bowl, where I knew he would have a drink of water, followed by a thorough and fastidious face washing.

FIRST AID FOR SEIZURES OR FITS

SEEK VETERINARY ATTENTION IMMEDIATELY
Most seizures require medical attention (especially if poisoning is
   suspected).
Get a diagnosis of the underlying cause.

CAUSES OF SEIZURES
Poisoning
Epilepsy
A blow to the head (concussion)
Colic, teething
Fevers

TYPES OF SEIZURES
Petit mal: small, brief episodes with subtle symptoms such as staring
   momentarily or experiencing short episodes of confusion

Grand mal: violent in appearance, escalating from a dazed look to frothing at the mouth and followed by collapse and violent shaking and thrashing

DURATION OF SEIZURES

Seizures may be several minutes in duration and subside gradually; alternatively, one convulsion may follow quickly after another.

Seizures that last more than five minutes or occur in a series are an *emergency. Seek veterinary attention immediately.*

WHAT TO DO

Remain calm.

Stay with the animal.

Remove collar from neck.

Clear area of sharp objects, electrical cords, etc.

Speak quietly and calmly and be reassuring.

If inside, darken the room with shades, curtains.

If outside, shield from sunlight or street light.

Call your veterinarian after the seizure is over.

If a seizure lasts more than five minutes, *seek veterinary attention immediately.*

WHAT NOT TO DO

Do not move the animal unnecessarily.

Do not put anything in the animal's mouth.

Do not hold the animal down.

Do not control the movements in any way.

Do not cover.

Do not shout or make loud noises.

Conditions that can cause, worsen, or escalate a seizure

   Bright or suddenly flashing lights (reflected sunlight).

   Sudden loud noises or explosions.

PREPARATIONS

Keep your vet's phone number handy.

For animals that have a history of seizures, make up a stock bottle of Nature's Rescue dilution to keep at hand: four to eight drops in a one-ounce bottle of distilled water. Take it everywhere the animal goes and place a few drops on the animal's lips at the first indication of a seizure coming on.

HOMEOPATHY FOR SEIZURES OR FITS

Status critical: *Seek veterinary attention immediately.* Give doses of four pellets at five- to ten-minute intervals en route to your veterinarian. Crush pillules in a piece of clean, folded paper and place powder between lip and gum.

Status acute: After an initial dose (four pellets), treatment may be repeated at fifteen-minute intervals for up to four doses or until condition is relieved; then consult your veterinarian. If there is no response, *seek veterinary attention immediately.*

SYMPTOMS	REMEDY
Seizures from fear or fright; acute, sudden, violent seizures; fits that begin as shaking of the head and dizziness; body cold; animal is fearful, anxious	Aconite (consider Nature's Rescue)
Seizures when fever is the cause; eyes staring, glassy; pupils dilated, sensitive to light; bleeding of the nose; dry mouth; violent tossing about	Bell
Seizures during teething or colic; symptoms begin as restlessness, snappishness, and impatience; involuntary diarrhea, hot, green, slimy stools; excessive drooling or salivation	Cham
Seizures associated with male hypersexuality or from fright, anticipatory fear, thunderstorms; excessive drooling or salivation; pupils dilated, insensitive to light; one pupil dilated, the other contracted; involuntary diarrhea; animal grabs out, is fearful of falling	Gels
Seizures—violent tremors everywhere; very tense scalp, oily sweat on head; foul smell to breath, excretions, and body; profuse perspiration; pale mucous membranes	Merc
Seizures with convulsions while conscious and worse from touch and movement;	Nux vom

convulsions brought on by great anger;
cramping—animal draws up the limbs;
sour perspiration on only one side of
the body; body hot, toes cold and blue

Seizures associated with male hypersexuality;   Phos
sudden seizures, prostration, faints;
causes: light, sound, excitement, touch,
thunderstorms; symptoms may begin as
dizziness with faintness; tongue dry,
smooth, red; animal usually lies on the
right side; numbness of forelegs and paws;
symptoms worse with touch, twilight,
thunderstorm, ascending stairs; symptoms
better in the dark

Initial stages of a seizure; remedy may slow a   Nature's Rescue*
seizure or prevent a series; may be used in
combination with other remedies

---

*Dilute four drops in an ounce of water and give four drops of this mixture on tongue
or lips (use a plastic eyedropper only). If animal is too agitated to give drops, flick
droplets into face; contact with any mucous membrane will allow remedy to cross
into the bloodstream. Or hold open bottle under nose, as with smelling salts.
Treatment may be repeated as needed until calm is restored.

CHAPTER 32

Shock

Shock results from physical or emotional trauma and is a symptom that is seen when the body attempts to provide adequate blood circulation to vital organs, such as the heart and brain, by automatically shutting down blood circulation to less vital areas of the body. Excessive blood loss from bleeding may also result from shock. Animals in shock are collapsed, the pulse is rapid and weak, breathing is rapid and shallow, and the skin is inelastic, with pale, dry mucous membranes of the mouth and eyes. Retention of body heat (or removal of excess body heat, as in the case of heatstroke) and adequate fluid intake are vital first-aid techniques. Veterinary attention to correct the cause and intravenous administration of appropriate fluids are recommended medical treatment for shock.

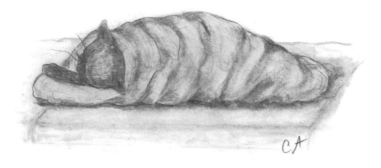

FIRST AID FOR SHOCK

If bleeding is severe, treat bleeding first. *Apply direct pressure.*
  Firmly press a clean, dry pad or cloth to the wound (if you have
    no pad, use your hand).
  Keep pressing firmly, enough to make bleeding stop. If pad
    becomes soaked, put a second pad on top of the first and press
    harder. *Do not* remove first pad—this interrupts clotting action.
  Keep pressing until bleeding stops or help is obtained.
  Raise bleeding part higher than the heart to slow bleeding.
Treat for shock. Cover the animal to retain body heat. You may use
  anything at hand: blankets, rugs, a sweater or coat, even newspa-
  pers or curtains.
Seek veterinary attention immediately.
Note: Shock is a serious medical emergency. More animals die from
  shock as the result of accident or injury than from any other
  cause. *Seek veterinary attention immediately.*

HOMEOPATHY FOR SHOCK

Status critical (shock with convulsions): *Seek veterinary attention
  immediately.* Give doses of four pellets at five- to ten-minute intervals en route to your veterinarian. Crush pillules in a piece of clean,
  folded paper and place powder between lip and gum.
Status acute: After an initial dose (four pellets), dosing may be
  repeated again in fifteen minutes. *Seek veterinary attention immediately.*

SYMPTOMS	REMEDY
Shock from extreme fright or trauma; restlessness and tossing about; mouth dry, tongue coated white; throat red, constricted	Aconite (consider Nature's Rescue)
Shock from extreme trauma, blows, falls; animal is very sore, resists touch	Arnica

Symptoms	Remedy
Shock with collapse; body icy cold, animal refuses to be covered; convulsions may occur	Camph
Shock from fear or anticipatory fear; animal is dizzy, drowsy, dull, trembling; great prostration, apathy	Gels
Shock from dehydration, loss of body fluids; eyes appear wet with tears; legs cold, pads perspiring	Nat mur (follow with electrolyte solution)
Symptoms the same as those of Aconite	Nature's Rescue*

*Dilute four drops in an ounce of water and give four drops of this mixture on tongue or lips. Repeat at five- to ten-minute intervals until animal responds more normally or until arrival at the veterinarian. If animal is unconscious, hold open bottle under the nose, as with smelling salts.

CHAPTER 33

Sprains and Strains

More often a situation involving older animals, strains and sprains usually result from overexertion and simple trauma. Nonetheless, overenthusiastic youngsters may also overdo or slip and fall. While restful recuperation is a must, single remedies, and sometimes remedies given in combination, will produce dramatic healing, as recounted in the following story.

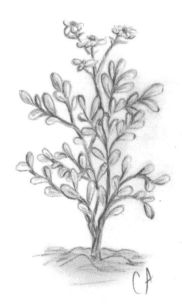

Rue Bitterwort

ARNICA, RHUS, AND RUTA FOR A SPRAIN

It was a mountain of paperwork. I'd not been looking forward to it, but it had to be done; my house was awash in piles of correspondence, forms, and case notes that needed sorting, answering, filling out, and filing. I sat at the round oak kitchen table shuffling through the piles, groping for inspiration from each stack I touched. Should I begin with this pile or that one? At my back, the sun beamed through the double windows, warming my shoulders, playfully beckoning me outdoors.

I could hear Hervena behind me in her rabbit hutch below the window, moving the flake of hay from one corner to the other. Without turning around and looking, I could tell from the sounds that she was grasping large bunches of hay in her mouth and carrying them to their new place. She often rearranged the contents of her hutch as though seeking to express a talent for interior design, a nesting instinct that fascinated and entertained me for hours at a time. She was busily at work, I realized with a guilty start, and I should follow her example.

Suddenly, a loud *thwack* reverberated in my ears, the unmistakable sound of a bird striking the windowpane behind me. Startled, I jerked my head around and saw the telltale gray breast feathers clinging to the outside of the glass; they fluttered gently in the rising heat, like fingers waving to attract my attention.

In a flash I was on my feet and out the back kitchen door. As I passed through the sunporch, a wall of hot air slowed me down, and I heard the shrill buzzing of a male cicada drumming the membranes on the side of his abdomen, announcing his emergence from nymphal case into the waiting world.

Outside, below the window, I found the blue jay huddled against the base of a burdock grown almost shrublike. His bright, deep blue feathers identified him as a male, and he trailed his right wing behind him as he sought refuge from my gaze behind the thick stalk. Now was the moment to gather him up, before he became so frightened by my presence that he tried to escape and further harmed himself. I reached between the heavy downy leaves, breaking a strand of spiderweb in doing so, and cupped my hands around him. His resistance was very faint, his struggles weak.

Back in the kitchen, I cast about for some type of small enclosure to place him in. I didn't have a birdcage; I preferred to enjoy watching the wild freedom of the various species of birds that sought refuge and food in my

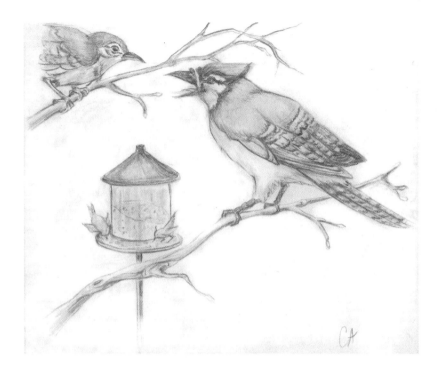

backyard. My eyes fell upon a yard-sale oddity left on the kitchen counter: a four- by four- by six-inch wire box, one side of which was a hinged door with a tiny clasp.

The wire was heavy gauge, almost an eighth of an inch in diameter, and spaced at three-quarter-inch intervals. I had no idea what it was originally intended to be used for and had bought it for fifty cents only because it was such an interesting curiosity. Now it became a made-to-order enclosure, which would enable me to safely house the injured blue jay. I tucked him inside, noting with a smile that the container was small enough to keep him from spreading his wings and further damaging his injured limb.

But there was a problem: all the sides were vertical wires; there were no horizontal wires that would serve as anchors for a perch. I rummaged around in a cabinet until I found a three-legged aluminum colander and a bamboo skewer. Placing the wire box in the bottom of the colander where it rested on its corners in the round base, I pushed the shaft of bamboo through the colander holes from one side to the other, making a perch that ran through the wire box about an inch from the bottom. The blue jay grasped the bamboo with his feet and sat on the makeshift perch, his feathers ruffled and his eyes squinted shut. I was pleased with my creativity, but I needed to turn my attention to the bird's injuries.

His wing hung limply at his side. I watched him a moment, taking in his stillness and wondering if he were going to go into shock. Warmth, Nature's Rescue, and Arnica all came to mind. I would begin by covering the small enclosure with a dish towel, to keep in the blue jay's body heat while I made up a dilution of Nature's Rescue.

He rustled a bit when I covered the wire box with the gingham cloth, but then he was still. I stirred four drops of Nature's Rescue tincture into an ounce of distilled water in a small glass, making an appropriate dilution for use. Because I knew that he would aspirate, breathing the liquid into his lungs, if I tried to give him drops by mouth, I squeezed a single drop from an eyedropper through the top of the box, aiming for his eye. It missed, ran down the side of his face, and landed on his chest, where it hung suspended, shimmering like a jewel against his pearly gray breast feathers. I tried again, and this time the drop landed on his eye, causing him to blink and wet his eye with the dilution. I waited and watched.

In less than a minute he opened his eyes and looked around. I must have looked huge to him, a gigantic face peering into his prison. Seeing me, he began to struggle for more secure footing on the bamboo skewer, perhaps trying to duck out of sight, as he had behind the burdock stem. His restlessness and anxiety were a very good sign. This was normal bird behavior that indicated that he was not going to die from the shock that claimed most bird's lives as the result of striking windowpanes.

I turned my attention to his wing. I noticed that he was trying to fold it up against his body. He flexed his shoulder muscles, and the wing began to fold up only to tremble and fall limply against his side again. I wondered if it were sprained and the muscles traumatized. As with the Nature's Rescue, I dissolved four pillules of Arnica 30c in another small glass of distilled water and aimed a drop at his eye. I was getting good with practice, and the drop found its appointed destination. Within a few minutes, he closed his eyes and tucked his beak into his chest feathers. I covered his enclosure with the gingham towel so he could sleep and went outside to begin my duties as a bird mother.

I would have to create a cache of food for him to eat during his confinement, whether his recovery time was one day or several. Birds need to eat a lot of insects in a twenty-four-hour period just to stay alive, and most of their moisture requirements come from their food. That meant that I would have to catch some pretty big and juicy bugs just to meet his minimal caloric and water requirements.

Over the next half hour I hunted bugs and placed them in several jars I had taken from the kitchen cabinet. It was not a task that appealed to me; I preferred furred, feathered, and finned animal companions over creepy-crawly acquaintances. My waiting pile of paperwork began to look more and more attractive with each grasshopper and beetle, and finally I could not bring myself to catch another insect. I went back inside the house to check on my new friend.

He was awake and surveying his surroundings. With tweezers I held out a grasshopper and, eyes squinted shut and teeth clenched, tried not to hear the sounds of him picking at the squirming morsel. I was grateful, when I opened my eyes, to see only the leg left between the tongs of the tweezers. That his appetite was intact was a very good sign that he would survive, and with newfound resolve, I offered him an earthworm, which he ignored. Perhaps he was full; perhaps he did not care for them. At any rate, it was time for him to rest, and after covering him again, I placed the jars in the refrigerator, where the captive dinners would be chilled to stillness and where I would not have to look at them.

Over the course of the day, I gave him several more drops of Arnica from the dilution that I had made up. Between doses, I offered lunch, a postlunch snack, predinner entree, dinner, and dessert. By eight in the evening, he was either full or not liking his menu choices, and I covered his enclosure with the setting of the summer sun. Dawn and his waking would come soon enough, and like any tired bird mother, I needed my rest, too.

I awoke to the sound of birdsong emanating from the kitchen and turned over in bed to see the first gray slivers of dawn streaking the sky outside my bedroom window. How glorious! Hervena was standing up on hind legs sniffing the air as I entered the kitchen; even she was enchanted with the melody that greeted the new day.

The jay, as I had come to think of him, was awake and sitting on his perch. His wing was folded against his side in a more normal position, held closer and higher to his body than the day before. Eyes bright and darting, he took in my movements toward him. As he began to edge away from my approach, I noticed that his movements were stiff and jerky. He was recovering; that much was evident by his energy and song. But he seemed stiff and lame this morning.

Morning stiffness always brought Rhus tox to mind, and I set about to mix up another remedy. While doing so, I wondered if the tendons and ligaments of his wing were also traumatized; this would indicate that Ruta graveolens would also be useful in his recovery. But were the other symptoms of Ruta also present? Yes, he was lame, but was he also weak with extreme lassitude? No, he did not exhibit lassitude; he did not seem limp in his body at all. But was he weak, or rather, was his wing weak? I decided to try a simple test to observe how he used or did not use his wing.

With tweezers, I secured a grasshopper from one of the jars in the refrigerator. Thankfully, it was chilled and did not offer any resistance as I poked it through the wires at the bottom of the enclosure. It lay there momentarily before beginning to move. As I suspected, the birdsong had been one of calling other birds and heralded the hunt for morning feeding. The jay spied the subtle movement under his perch and craned his neck to investigate.

As he leaned out over the bamboo perch, he lost his balance and instinctively lifted both wings to catch himself. Although there was not enough room within the enclosure to fully spread either of his wings, his uninjured wing opened and closed with ease. The right wing moved almost imperceptibly and drooped, hanging weakly as it had the day before. He regained his balance by lifting his head and peered at the wriggling grasshopper below.

This was all the evidence I needed to make my remedy choices. I knew from experience that all three remedies (Arnica, Rhus tox, and Ruta) are symbiotic in healing trauma to muscles, ligaments, and tendons, especially when weakness and stiffness are accompanying symptoms. It was very likely that all components of the jay's wing were affected by the accident; the muscles were probably bruised, ligaments and tendons likely strained. I also knew that these were three remedies that I could mix together in one dilution, without worry that any one would act as an antidote to either of the others. Using them together would address all the injuries to his wing and speed healing.

But he needed to have breakfast first. Birds use up most of their calorie reserves overnight keeping warm, and the morning feeding is the most important to all species. To replenish their spent calories, birds have to eat the equivalent of their body weight as near dawn as possible. If they do not, their metabolism winds down like a clock, their heart rate and circulatory system slow, and with lowered body temperature, they become chilled and soon die.

Into the jar and back into the refrigerator went the jumping grasshopper. It was too early in the morning for me to cope with wriggling insects. After consuming four crickets, six lady bugs, and two black beetles, the jay began to preen his wing feathers. Hervena took advantage of the quiet interlude to vie for my attention. She was hopping back and forth in her hutch, indicating that she would like some crunchy burdock root and dandelion greens for her breakfast. After feeding her and filling her water bottle with fresh spring water, I sat back to enjoy a steaming cup of tea and watch the dawn unfold.

By nine o'clock, I had given the jay two drops of the mixture of Arnica, Rhus tox, and Ruta dissolved together in the same glass of distilled water. The jay slept the morning away, making soft rustling noises as I bent to the task of my paperwork. Soon it was time for his lunch, and I steeled myself to the task of hand-feeding him. But he ate well and with an enthusiasm that made my job easier; I could tell with relief that he was no longer stiff and weak.

The day wore quietly on. Pile after pile of paperwork was conquered. I took a couple of calls from people with animal companions who had various symptoms: a cat whose symptoms indicated Hepar for an abscess and a puppy with yellow ear discharges that would respond to Pulsatilla nigricans. Replacing the telephone receiver in its cradle, I decided that the next morning would be a good time to decide if the jay was recovered enough to be released. Tomorrow I would give him a good breakfast so that he would not have to hunt for insects and could rest his wing for most of the day. If he was no longer stiff and lame, and if he held his wing at a normal posture, I would perhaps release him. Perhaps.

That night, I gave him another drop of the remedy mixture and went to bed, looking forward to the new day with as much excitement as I had eagerly awaited Christmas morning as a child. But when morning came, I realized that he was not ready; he still did not move his wing with the strength I felt was necessary to sustain flight. I decided that I would give him four doses of the remedy mixture each day until he recovered.

His release came two days later. I had restocked the insect larder twice and was becoming used to hand-feeding him. That final dawn, when I fed him his last meal, he was nervous and jumpy and moved around restlessly in the confinement of his small enclosure. Fifteen minutes after feeding him the last grasshopper, I gave him one last dose of the remedy mixture. It was time.

With mixed emotions I carried his enclosure out to the back steps. Once outside, he became alive with motion, turning his head back and forth with each trill of birdsong that came from the woods around the house. He was ready, and so must I be. I pulled at the clasp that held the small door closed and opened it wide; he leaned far out and, bobbing his head, jumped to the railing. In a flash of blue, he was gone.

I stood in the morning stillness, hearing the cicadas buzzing in the gathering heat. The sound reminded me of the last jar of insects that I had taken from the refrigerator, which now lay at my feet. It was release day for them, too. I opened the jar and spilled them onto the stoop, where they lay and sat in the sudden heat, gathering warmth and strength enough to make their escape.

Startled, I stepped back as a whoosh of wings beat the air in front of the railing; it was the jay. In one deft swoop, he dived toward the insects at my feet and streaked away toward the spruce at the edge of the clearing. I saw him there for only a second before he took wing, the sun coming up behind him making a silhouette of his form with the grasshopper dangling from his beak.

FIRST AID FOR SPRAINS AND STRAINS

TYPES OF SPRAINS, FROM LEAST TO MOST SERIOUS
Simple sprains
> A temporary displacement of two opposite joint surfaces and a
>   partial tearing of the adjacent ligaments that surround the joint
Sprains complicated by laceration of ligaments
> Sprains that include complete tearing of ligaments surrounding a
>   joint
Sprains complicated by avulsion of bone
> Also called sprain fracture—a simple sprain complicated by a

fragment of bone torn loose along with a partial tear of ligaments surrounding a joint

HOME CARE OF SPRAINS AND STRAINS
Reduce swelling and heat by application of cold packs or cloths.
Immobilize animals by confinement in a small pen or box.
Choose a homeopathic remedy from the list and give according to frequency of dosage instructions.
Seek veterinary attention and treatment if discomfort lasts more than two days.

HOMEOPATHY FOR SPRAINS AND STRAINS

Status acute: After an initial dose (four pellets), treatment may be repeated at one- to two-hour intervals for up to four doses or until condition is relieved. If no relief is obtained, consult your veterinarian.

Status chronic: After an initial dose (four pellets), continue with two doses a day or until symptoms subside. If symptoms do not subside, consult your veterinarian.

SYMPTOMS	REMEDY
Sprains/strains with bruising	Arnica
Sprains/strains with morning stiffness, overuse of muscles in damp weather	Rhus tox
Sprains/strains with tendon/ligament involvement; extreme lassitude, lameness, weakness	Ruta

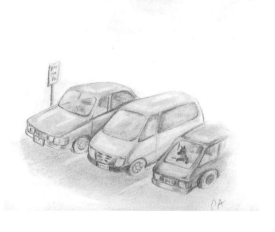

CHAPTER 34

Sunburn and Heatstroke

We rarely think that if our dogs are out in their pens or tied to their doghouses on a sunny summer day, they may be candidates for sunburns. But like humans, all animals are susceptible to overexposure to the sun. Be sure that your animal companion has shade available to him or her as well as plenty of fresh drinking water.

We all know that the inside of cars and other vehicles gets dangerously hot on summer days, right? Still, animal control agents are called to countless parking lots each summer to rescue dogs confined in vehicles. What is a few minutes in the supermarket to you may be a life-threatening situation for your dog if left in a car on a warm, sunny day. The cardinal rule is *don't*.

A LUCKY DOG

It was the fourth day in a row of hot, sultry August weather on the coast of Maine. Not a breeze stirred, not a puff of salt air wafted in from the bay. Like many other people, I had used the excuse to do a bit of shopping, to seek a brief respite in the air-conditioned coolness of the supermarket. A half hour of wandering around up and down the aisles produced little of interest; I bought toothpaste, organic carrots, and, impulsively, a bright beach towel. But it was thirty minutes of welcomed respite from the stifling heat of temperatures in the upper nineties, and feeling somewhat revived, I made my way to the parking lot.

I was just getting into my car when I heard the weak bark come from the truck parked beside my car. I looked but saw no dog, and I thought that the heat had fired my imagination. Opening my own car door too wide, I bumped the truck beside me with its edge, and a brown head appeared at the bottom of the truck's passenger-side window. I turned and looked. Glassy black eyes stared back at me. Front paws scrabbled for a purchase, the brown head wobbled, lurched, and was suddenly gone. I looked at the top of the truck window; it was rolled down a scant two inches, and shimmers of heat rose above the truck roof.

With the outside temperature over ninety-five degrees, and the truck sitting in full sunlight in an open, unshaded parking lot, it must have been well over 100 degrees inside the truck. In alarm I reached for the door handle of the truck. It was locked, and so was the driver's side door. I knew that the truck hadn't been there when I had arrived, so the dog inside hadn't been in distress for more than half an hour. But I also knew that on a summer day temperatures in a car can reach 120 degrees in a matter of minutes, whether it is parked in the shade or not, and even short-term exposure to high temperatures, when combined with lack of ventilation, can lead to permanent brain damage.

Standing on tiptoe, I spied the dog lying on the floor panel, panting and gasping for breath where he had sought the coolest part of the confining space. Heat rises, and I knew that he was a very lucky dog to have been seen the first time; he probably wouldn't get up onto the seat again. There was no time to lose; seconds were precious and could mean life or death in this situation. Almost without thinking, I reached into my car and pressed the horn and kept pressing.

Two women were passing and stopped to ask what I was doing. I quickly explained, forcing my voice to carry evenly and calmly. I would need my wits about me, and many things would need to fall into place so I could help this dog. I urgently needed the help of these two bystanders, and the errands that I was about to send them on needed to be explained calmly and clearly.

Within moments they returned. One carried a bag of ice and a disposable paper take-out food bucket filled with water. The other had arranged for the store manager to announce over the intercom system that the truck's owner was wanted in the parking lot. As backup, in case the owner was elsewhere, she had also called the local police to send an officer to the scene at once.

Five minutes went by. An eternity. With my hands, I forced the truck window down another inch and talked to the dog. He lay there on the floor, not responding. Another two minutes went by and my heart was sinking. A police cruiser pulled up and an officer I knew jumped out. Within seconds he had the truck door open. He placed the dog on a grassy median strip behind the truck and stood back. The dog stood there uncertainly for a moment—weak, trembling, and gasping for breath. He was staring with a glassy expression that indicated a dull stupor, his lips and mouth bright red. Suddenly he began to vomit and have diarrhea simultaneously. Then he collapsed.

The officer leaped into action, instructing the two women to put the ice into the bucket of water and asking me if I had a towel or blanket. My heart leaped for joy! Here was one of my town's finest, and he did not hesitate to use his first-aid skills on a dog! Together we wet down the dog, beginning with his head and mouth. Cold water applied to the head and mouth will bring body temperature down quickly. We soaked my beach towel in water and applied it to the dog's head, neck, and back, placing ice cubes under it, in places where they might stay put for a few minutes. I knelt down and began rubbing the dog's mouth, tongue, and gums with a piece of ice, to

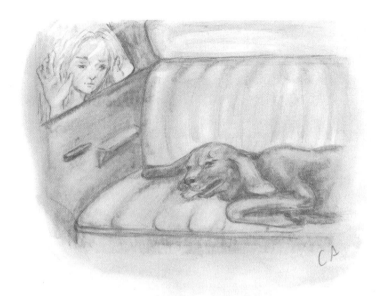

further speed the cooling process. In my hands I could feel waves of heat coming from his body, and his head lolled from side to side. He had lost consciousness but was twitching restlessly. Both his body and his brain were overheated. I was concerned that convulsions were not far behind.

At this, the officer seemed to become convinced that the dog might not pull through. I had put the small homeopathic kit from my car in my purse, not wanting to leave it in the baking heat of the glove compartment, and I now pulled it out. "I have some first-aid homeopathic remedies," I began. "I have one in particular that really might help, if you think it would be appropriate to give it in the owner's absence and without his permission."

This, I knew, was a legal matter. To medically tend someone's animal companion in their absence and without their permission was questionable at best. Still, I hoped that the officer would grasp at my proffered straw and acquiesce to this minor indiscretion. If he gave me permission to do so, I could act without hesitation. And the owner had left the dog in a life-threatening situation and should have known better. Wasn't any necessary intervention appropriate in this case?

"We've got to do something," the officer agreed. "Whatever you've got that might help, use it. Quickly. Whoever owns this dog has given up their rights as an animal owner as far as I'm concerned." He seemed upset, as though his concern had finally given way to anger. "They won't have much to say about anything when I get hold of them."

I wasn't sure if I should put the pillules of Belladonna 30c in his cheek pouch; he was still unconscious, and I was concerned that he might choke, especially if he began to convulse. And I had nothing in which to mix them. Improvise, I thought. There were the dredges of melted ice water in the paper bucket, and I mixed the pillules in there. No eyedropper. Improvise again, I thought. The dog's twitching had not escalated into convulsions, and for this I was grateful; I bent the edge of the paper bucket into a spout and poured a couple of drops onto his lips.

While I waited I checked his physical status. His pulse was quick and faint; his breathing was heavy, quick, and coming in irregular puffs; and his pupils were quite dilated. I watched his eye, holding one lid open a few seconds at a time, because pupil constriction, back to a normal size, is an indication that Belladonna is working. Within a few minutes his pupils resumed a more normal size, and his breath became less labored and more even. For me, the few minutes seemed interminably long, yet he was in a very critical state. To see his symptoms recede within a few minutes was nothing less than a miracle.

I gave him another two doses, a few drops on the lips at five-minute intervals, and he soon came around. He still looked dazed and shaky, seeming to wonder where he was and why he was covered with a wet towel and surrounded by strangers. I soothed him as best I could, trying to be brave myself and attempting to make my voice sound comforting and positive. This was difficult for me, since I knew that he had experienced a close brush with death and might still suffer long-term effects of brain damage from being overheated. I looked at the positive aspects of the situation. He was a lucky dog to have four strangers trying to save his life, one of whom just happened to have a homeopathic first-aid kit in her purse.

By this time the woman who had brought water the first time had returned with another bucket of water. I had asked her to retrieve the restaurant packets of salt and sugar I had stashed in my glove compartment, and together we mixed up a crude electrolyte solution. As he lay in the grass, the dog drank willingly from the bucket, short laps at first, then more enthusiastically. He still had far to go, but it was a very positive response, and my anxiety lessened slightly. The officer returned to his car to answer a radio call from a vet that had been transferred through a dispatcher. We anxiously watched the dog and waited for his owner to show up.

In a moment the officer returned and scooped up the dog in his arms. "The vet at Bayview Animal Clinic has agreed to see him and keep him for further treatment, if necessary," the officer said, speaking to the three of us, who had been staying with the dog. "It's possible that he has seen this dog before and knows the owner.

"I want to thank each of you for acting quickly and calmly. Your actions probably saved the life of this dog, and if he's very lucky, he will recover fully. We get several calls like this each summer, and for the life of me I can't understand why people leave animals in cars in any weather. I've also known people to leave their children alone in circumstances like this, and I don't understand that either." He turned and put the dog on the front seat of his car and climbed in after him.

I watched them drive away and sent my prayers after them. I would call my vet, Marc, later that evening and ask how the dog was doing. It was another of those interesting coincidences, that this dog was on his way to the clinic that met all of my own animals' health care needs.

Later, after a light dinner, I sat on the back porch, where a slight breeze had picked up. I took the telephone out with me and called Marc. "He's doing well," he told me. "I've had him on intravenous fluids all day, and he had a bit of dinner a while ago. No, I don't think he's going to have any lasting damage as the result of his experience, but a few more minutes in that truck would have had a very different outcome."

I asked about the dog's owner and if he had been found. "I can't reveal the person's name because of confidentiality, but he was found and notified. As soon as we called, he came in to see how his dog was doing. He was very worried; he thought that his dog had been stolen. Apparently, he had taken his little girl into the clothing store next door to return a dress, and she tripped over a display stand and sprained her ankle. That's what kept him so long and why no one could find him. I advised him that leaving his dog home when he went on shopping trips would be much more comfortable for everyone—especially his dog," Marc added as an afterthought.

All in all, it had been a very good day. Everything had turned out all right. But I had one last question. I wanted a name that I could put with my image of that dog, a name that I could say in my prayers that night before going to sleep.

"The dog's name?" asked Marc. "His name is Lucky Dog."

FIRST AID FOR
SUNBURN AND HEATSTROKE

Heatstroke occurs in all species of animals. It may be caused by exposure of an animal's body to high temperatures, high humidity, and inadequate ventilation or by doing hard work in intense heat. *Never* leave your animal in a car—even with the windows open—on any day, summer or winter. On a summer day, temperatures in a car can reach 120 degrees in a matter of minutes. You must treat heatstroke immediately.

SYMPTOMS OF HEATSTROKE
Weakness
Muscle tremors
Panting and increased pulse rate
Collapse
Staring expression, vomiting, diarrhea, a bright red mouth, and elevated body temperature

FIRST AID FOR HEATSTROKE
Move to a cool, well-ventilated, and shaded area.
Apply cold water to the body.
Follow with electrolyte solution.
Seek veterinary attention immediately.

FIRST AID FOR SUNBURNS (TREAT AS FOR SECOND-DEGREE BURNS)
Submerge or rinse in cold water or apply cloths soaked in cold water.
If blisters are closed, apply clean bandage.
If blisters are open, *do not* cover.
Do not break blisters or peel skin.
Let heal naturally.
If burn is extensive or does not heal, consult your veterinarian.

HOMEOPATHY FOR
SUNBURN AND HEATSTROKE

Status critical: *Seek veterinary attention immediately.* Give doses of four pellets at five- to ten-minute intervals en route to your veterinarian.
Status acute: After an initial dose (four pellets), dosing may be

repeated at fifteen-minute intervals for up to four doses or until relief is obtained. If there is no response, *seek veterinary attention immediately.*

Status chronic (as in sunburn pain): After an initial dose (four pellets), treatment may be repeated at half-hour intervals for up to four doses or until condition is relieved. If there is no response, consult your veterinarian.

SYMPTOMS	REMEDY
First remedy to consider for heatstroke or severe sunburns; suddenness of symptoms; skin: red, hot, swollen, dry, burning; animal is faint, prostrate, anxious	Aconite (consider Nature's Rescue and follow with electrolyte solution*)
Heatstroke or severe sunburns; nausea, vomiting; dull stupor, heavy, hot; thirstlessness and restlessness	Bell (follow with electrolyte solution)
Minor sunburns, itchy; cold relieves but increases inflammation	Canth
Heatstroke or severe sunburns; animal is dizzy, drowsy, dull, and trembling; loss of muscle control, limpness; collapse, prostration; slow pulse	Gels (follow with electrolyte solution)
Symptoms the same as aconite	Nature's Rescue (follow with electrolyte solution)†

*See recipe in Appendix.

†Dilute four drops in an ounce of water and give four drops of this mixture on tongue or lips. Or hold open bottle under nose, as with smelling salts. Treatment may be repeated as needed until calm is restored or until arrival at the veterinarian.

CHAPTER 35

Surgery

Almost all surgery in veterinary practice is necessary to preserve life, alleviate suffering, or reduce the number of unwanted offspring, as in the case of spaying and neutering. However necessary or minor, surgery is considered in homeopathic terms a trauma to the body. Trauma may be perceived by the surgical candidate as either physical or emotional, and frequently as both. Do consider the remedies Aconite and Arnica in all surgical situations. When used according to the following instructions, recovery from surgical procedures is rapid and uneventful.

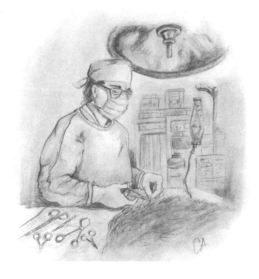

LILY'S SECOND CHANCE

It wasn't even a break in the bone or cartilage. It was a simple dislocated elbow. I could see that from the radiograph I held in my hand. How this old girl had walked on it for the past two days was beyond me. She lay on the backseat of the station wagon, waiting for less than a minute for me to come out of the clinic. Wet snowflakes pelted my face and the film that dangled from a paper clip and fluttered in the wind, leaving wet streaks on both.

My friend Sand who worked at the local animal shelter had called me the night before. The police had seen the old dog get hit by a car and had transported her to the nearest vet clinic less than a mile away. But there was a problem. Neither the city nor the shelter wanted to pick up the vet expenses for such an old dog, and it was considered more cost-effective to have her euthanized. When Sand learned this, she contacted me to intervene; I picked Lily up at the clinic moments before she was scheduled to be euthanized.

"Lily!" I screamed, climbing into the front seat. That was what Sand had decided to call her—lilies, white ones, being big, beautiful spring flowers that usher in a time of rebirth for all things that sheltered from and survive the cold days and long, dark nights of a New England winter. We were going to give her a second chance, another spring, and with our help her new season was soon to begin. I screamed not because she was in trouble, lying there patiently waiting for me, but because she was stone-deaf. I wasn't sure that she could hear me at all, but I shouted anyway. "I'll have you there in no time!" I shouted again. "Here we go!"

On the ride to Marc's clinic the storm picked up fiercely. Wet tar quickly turned into ice patches, and our pace slowed to compensate. My thoughts turned to my conversation with Sand the night before. I had wanted to know if anyone had a clue as to where she came from and what her condition was when Sand had first seen her.

"The police think that she's just been wandering around for quite some time. She's very thin; I don't think she's eaten for quite a few days." Sand's voice sounded faint over the telephone lines. "They think that she just wandered off from somewhere and nobody noticed. You should see how absolutely filthy she is; I don't think she's had a bath in years, and with that kind of neglect, I'm not surprised that whoever owned her didn't notice she was missing. Or care to notice," she added sadly.

"They also told me that they saw her just wander into the path of the oncoming car. The people who hit her were quite upset. It wasn't their fault, and they tried to stop, but with the new snow on the road, they slid right into her. I think that she was dizzy and faint from hunger. She's also totally deaf, and given her very old age, she probably doesn't see very well either. That would account for her lack of reaction; I don't think she saw or heard the car at all. It probably saved her life that she wasn't all tensed up with fear when the car ran into her."

A whimper and a thump from the backseat jolted me out of my reverie. I looked in the rearview mirror, craning my neck, but did not see Lily anywhere. She's fallen on the floor, I thought with dismay, pulling over to the side of the road.

Opening the car door, I saw her struggling on the floorboards. Wind carried wet, cold snow into the car as I reached in and lifted her back up onto the seat. Outwardly, it didn't seem to faze her much, falling and being moved. But I knew better; she was just very old, couldn't hear, and probably couldn't see. I wondered whether her vocal cords were likewise affected by her age and whether she *could* bark to indicate that she was in pain. Things would get better in a short time, I thought resolutely, climbing back into the front seat and gripping the steering wheel again.

Marc's only comment was "Wow." And he said it in a rather subdued voice. I wasn't sure if his restrained tone was a reaction to her physical condition or in astonishment at her odor. Bless his heart, he picked her up in his arms and carried her out back. I followed, quietly, the streaked and spotted radiograph dangling from its paper clip in my hand.

He looked at me over Lily's form stretched out on the exam table and reached silently for the film. I waited, holding my breath. "What's her name?" he asked noncommittally. I told him, resting a protective hand on Lily's shoulder. Was it to comfort her or to reassure me? I wondered. Marc studied the film for another long moment. I had never seen him look so stern and could not understand why. Finally, he broke the tension.

"She's lucky. It's a dislocated elbow and nothing more. Easy to fix, and it'll heal rapidly. But she's old. Who will take her? Have you given this a lot of thought? As much as you should?" His gaze was even and serious.

I smiled. "We've anchored a foster home for her while we find a permanent adoptive home. Sand has already established a financial fund for her; she's calling it the "Lily Fund." And one of her friends is sponsoring a dance to raise funds for her vet bills, food, and other care."

Marc grinned widely, "Thought so," he said, quickly covering up his soft response with another firm and even look. "Petra's spending the day at home with her cat, Jake, who's recovering from his neutering. You're appointed to help." The injection of sedative was given quickly, and Lily lay snoozing on the table a few minutes later. Tying the surgical gown behind my back, I wondered why Marc would have me put one on. I didn't have long to wait to find out.

"You need to lean over her right shoulder and hold her upper foreleg completely immobile." Marc pointed to the steel exam table. I leaned over and grasped Lily just below the shoulder, looking down at her snoring under my chest. The unmistakable odor of skunk assailed my nostrils and stung my eyes. Now why hadn't I noticed it before?

Marc took up his position in front of Lily and opposite me and studied the radiograph clipped to the illuminated screen on the wall across the room. "Hold," he said in a commanding voice, placing both hands around Lily's forearm just below the elbow. He pulled. He pulled more. He pulled a bit more, crescents of sweat beads materializing across his forehead. I watched, fascinated, as Lily's leg stretched and stretched, beyond a point I'd thought possible. Infeasible as it seemed, Marc pulled even more, and the leg stretched impossibly further. I could hear a creaking noise, much like floorboards squeaking; Marc twisted the foreleg slightly and released. The long lower bone snapped neatly into place, restoring the limb to its proper length.

"Let go and stand back a bit, please. You did great. Now I want to see if it's in the right place and not beside where it's supposed to be." He took Lily's wrist and gently flexed the foreleg back and forth. It worked with a fluid movement, like any sturdy hinge. Sweat dripped from his curly dark hair down his temple and into the crease in front of his ear. "Now we'll apply a soft elbow cast," he said, wiping the trickle away with the back of his hand.

Over the wrist and tugged onto the re-placed elbow joint went the soft cloth cast. Marc used surgical tape to tighten it and a few wraps to tape it top and bottom, above and below the joint. While he worked, he gave me instructions.

"She needs to stay off it for the rest of the day. She'll need help going to the bathroom, but that's the only time I want her up for the next twenty-four hours. And I want you, or whoever is going to take care of her, to support her weight when she is standing. This joint needs rest in order to heal, and it shouldn't have any weight on it until tomorrow.

"It's fine for her to eat and drink lying down for the next few days, too. But that's nothing to think about until after dinner tonight; the sedative won't wear off for another few hours, and she might be nauseous and not want to eat right away anyway. When she does wake up, she can have a very little drink, not more than a couple of laps—just enough to wet her tongue. And no baths, not until this elbow cast comes off. No matter how bad she smells!"

Marc carried Lily to the station wagon and placed her on the backseat for me. "I'll have Petra send you the bill. And here's a packet of mild pain relievers if she is uncomfortable. I know you well enough to know that you might choose to give her homeopathic remedies instead, but here they are in case you decide to use them." He pressed a small packet into my hand and squeezed my fingers around the bundle. "Be careful driving," he said, releasing my hand. "If Petra stays away any longer, I just might have to call you to come in and help me again."

The drive to Sand's house was quiet; the plows and sand trucks had already traveled most of my route to her driveway. Snow fell less and less, the flakes crystallizing in the dropping temperatures, and the driving was no longer slippery and treacherous. Lily slept all the way, and I drove slowly and easily through the white winter landscape, sparkling red, gold, and mauve in the setting sun.

We removed her from the backseat using the blanket she'd lain on as a stretcher. Sand had arranged a cushioned pen for her in the living room opposite the woodstove. It was enclosed by a folding child's gate arranged in a half circle, fastened on one side to the door frame leading to the kitchen and on the other to a heavy wing chair. Here Lily would be safe and confined from wandering when she was not being watched. We sat on the floor beside the pen, our homeopathic kits open before us, and watched Lily continue her sleep.

"There's a bunch of remedies that will be helpful to her," I began. "We probably have all the ones we need between us. Let's see." I began rummaging around in the big gray fishing tackle box I kept my remedies in. "She needs several when she first wakes up. But we should give them in the reverse order of her injuries. We should resolve the most recent trauma first, peel away the layers as it were."

Sand sat opposite me, legs crossed under her, pencil poised over the pad of paper she'd picked up before we sat down. She wrote the list while I recited the injuries and the corresponding remedies.

"The last trauma that she experienced was the surgery, pulling on her leg to relocate the joint. Arnica would be good for the bruising and trauma to all the structures in and around the elbow joint. If she seems frightened at all when she wakes up, we might assume that the surgery was frightening, and Aconite would be indicated in this first group of remedies. The sedative came before that, so Ledum for the needle puncture and Phosphorus to help her system discharge any remaining drug—but only after she wakes up. The sedative is a good thing right now; it's helping her sleep and acts as a pain reliever, too."

Sand looked up from her writing. "I've never dislocated anything, but I'll bet it hurts," she said, looking over at Lily. "Poor thing," she added, shaking her head. "I'm glad we rescued her." A small smile played at the corners of her mouth and lit up her eyes. I was glad, too.

"The accident itself was before that," I continued. "Bruising, fear, trauma to muscles and possibly bones, for sure to the tendons, ligaments, and the elbow joint cartilage. So, in order, we have more Arnica, Aconite, Arnica again, and Hypericum. Wow, that's quite a list," I said, leaning over and looking at Sand's neat writing.

"And a lot of Arnica," Sand noted. I nodded in agreement. "That's probably the most important remedy for her of all of them. I'll bet that's the one she'll need last, too."

We went through our kits, pulling out the five bottles. We decided to use 30c potencies for all the remedies. Sand thought it would be good to give Lily the Arnica when she woke up. We decided that she would follow that with single doses of the remedies in the order they appeared on the list: Aconite, Ledum, Phosphorus, Arnica, Aconite, Arnica, and Hypericum, giving them in single doses. If she napped after taking any remedy, Sand would wait until she woke before giving her the next one. If Lily didn't nap, Sand would wait a couple of hours before giving the next remedy. This was somewhat different from the usual way we gave remedies to animals in our care, and Sand mentioned it.

"It's called sequential homeopathy. I read about it in a book by a Dutch homeopath; he wrote that healing layers of trauma, beginning with the most recent, completely cured many injuries. Even historical symptoms—

from very old injuries that happened long ago. I've tried it in a few cases that I've taken, and it works." We agreed that this was a pretty good plan, and I made my preparations to leave for home. We would be in touch by phone over the next few days to discuss how Lily's story continued to unfold.

Sand called mid-morning to fill me in on Lily's progress. "It was very interesting to watch her respond to each remedy; I wouldn't have believed it unless I was there myself."

"What do you mean?" I asked.

"Well, when she woke up, I took her out. And when she came back in, she had a small drink of water. Then I started giving her the remedies. She fell back to sleep right after the first one, Arnica. She woke up twenty minutes later, and she seemed really scared. So then I gave her the Aconite, and she fell asleep almost immediately. That time, she slept only ten minutes or so, but when she woke, she seemed dizzy and woozy. I figured it was time for the Phosphorus, and gave her the single dose. But she didn't fall asleep, instead she whined in pain. I touched her leg, moving up and down over the length, trying to figure out where it hurt. Know what I found?" she asked triumphantly.

"What?"

"Her leg didn't hurt at all. It was the muscle over her shoulder blade, where she had had the sedative injection. I realized that the remedies were healing all her traumas in the reverse order of their original occurrence, and as each remedy worked the next layer of symptoms was surfacing. This is really amazing!"

"Then what?" I wanted to know.

"Well, the Ledum didn't make her sleepy at all, and I thought that it didn't work. But then she got up and changed position. It seemed that she just couldn't get comfortable. She started to get really restless, but she seemed so heavy, as if any movement was like trying to lift a great weight. I remembered when Buddy sprained his leg last fall, and he had the same symptoms—we used Arnica, remember?"

"Uh-huh," I murmured.

"I looked at the list, and Arnica was next!"

"So how did it work?"

"She's still sleeping. I'll give her Hypericum later, if her elbow is sensitive to touch, and more doses of Arnica, too, maybe one or two a day, if she seems sore while she is healing. I wouldn't have believed any of this unless I had seen it for myself," Sand said again.

It was truly amazing. Symptom after symptom had resolved, followed immediately by the appearance of the one previous to it. It was like peeling layers of an onion. I had never expected the remedies to work so quickly, but then everything that had happened to Lily over the past two days had happened quickly. And the next ten days were no less miraculous for her.

She was adopted by Gabe, a woman who lived alone, and was immediately drawn into the web of Gabe's life, where she became as one who had been waited for. Gabe had a small cabin, warm, comfortable, and deep in the stillness of the Maine woods. No traffic threatened outside; the fireplace was equipped with a full-size screen; and Gabe's resident cat, Maxwell, took an immediate and proprietary liking to Lily. Evenings, he and she curled up at Gabe's feet while she read by the light of kerosene lamps, and they slept together near the hearth each night as the Maine winter gave way to the lilies that came with spring.

She appeared out of nowhere, a castoff with an unknown past. It was no less than miraculous that we had found out about her and had acted with the blind courage of faith that she could be and was worth saving, despite what many others had thought. The one good year that I hoped she'd have has given way to two, and I suspect that Gabe's and Maxwell's love will sustain her for a few more yet.

FIRST AID FOR SURGERY

INDICATIONS AND POSSIBLE CAUSES OF POSTSURGICAL COMPLICATIONS

Repeated vomiting
> Suspect infection or anesthesia withdrawal problems.

Dizziness, disorientation, dilated pupils in normal light, lasting more than twenty-four hours after arriving home
> Suspect anesthesia withdrawal problems.

Fever, excess body heat, or sweats
> Always suspect infection.

Tenderness, heat, and swelling of the incision site
Always suspect infection.

WHAT TO DO

If infection is suspected, consult your veterinarian and follow his or
her instruction.

Provide good nursing care.
A quiet, restful environment
Adequate nutrition
Assistance, as necessary, with eating, bowel and bladder elimina-
tion, and grooming

Choose from one of the homeopathic remedies listed and follow
instructions for dosage frequency.

If no response is seen after a few doses, consult your veterinarian.

HOMEOPATHY FOR SURGERY

Status critical: *Seek veterinary attention immediately.* Give doses of four
pellets at five- to ten-minute intervals en route to your veterinarian.

Status acute: After an initial dose (four pellets), dosing may be
repeated at one- to two-hour intervals for up to four doses or until
condition is relieved. If there is no response, consult your veterinarian.

Status chronic: After an initial dose (four pellets), continue with two
doses a day or until symptoms subside. If there is no response, consult your veterinarian.

SYMPTOMS	REMEDY
Any surgical pain with fear before or after surgery	Aconite (consider Nature's Rescue)
Bruising, soreness from surgery	Arnica
After bone, nerve surgery; site very sensitive to touch	Hyper

| Postoperative vomiting from anesthesia; aids body in secreting anesthesia | Phos (follow with electrolyte solution) |
| Similar to Aconite symptoms | Nature's Rescue* |

*Dilute four drops in an ounce of water and give four drops of this mixture on tongue or lips. Or hold open bottle under the nose, as with smelling salts. Treatment may be repeated as needed until calm is restored or until the arrival at your veterinarian.

CHAPTER 36

Teeth Injuries

Contrary to popular belief, many injuries to companion animals' teeth can be remedied by your veterinarian. Such skills may be part of your veterinarian's repertoire, or he or she may refer you to another vet well-practiced in veterinary dentistry. An unusual story follows, one that I hope will warm your heart and make you smile.

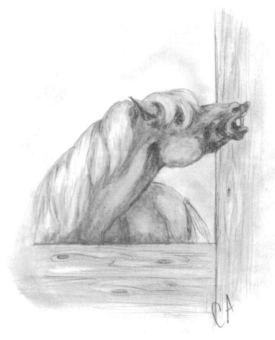

LEAPIN' GUINEA PIGS!

Amnesia teetered and tottered at the edge of the hassock, holding on with her tiny claws to the very edge of the small braided rug tacked to the cushion. The tuft of hair that stood up on the top of her head puffed out, giving her a comical appearance. She was a guinea pig with medium-length multicolored hair in tones of rust brown, black, and white. She had several swirls in her coat where the hair parted and lay in fans clockwise against the grain; these, along with her coat of many colors, lent her overall appearance a hint of court jester persona. She was the first guinea pig ever to live with me and was named by her previous family as a sort of joke. ("What did you say her name was?" "I can't remember!")

We spent lots of time together, she and I, and varied were her playgrounds. Although her enclosure was big enough to house fifty guinea pigs, well-equipped and comfortable, she preferred to be with me most of the time. We went to the store together, she riding hidden in the pocket of my jacket; in the car she nested in the glove compartment, held securely in place by a small window screen that replaced the hinged cover. The third drawer of my desk was another of her favorite places to play when I was working at my writing; this was closest to the floor and notched out on the side, which allowed her the freedom to climb in and out. She had the run of the house, which I had quickly guinea pig–proofed upon her arrival: all electrical cords were securely anchored high up on walls with duct tape, low electrical outlets inserted with child-proofing plugs, entrances behind appliances and to small rodent-sized curiosities closed off from her ever-inquisitive explorations. If there was a Guinea Pig Heaven, she had found it, and it was a deep source of delight and honor for me to provide her with it.

Still, of all the world she had to roam, her favorite place was the hassock at my feet as I watched the evening news. Often she would sit there quietly, sometimes exploring my stockinged feet on one side and at other times scurrying along the perimeter to peer from up on high at the world below. I think that she liked it so much because the height gave her a visual vista that was a new perspective to her, being at floor level most of the time.

The evening of the accident she was engaged in a particular acrobatic maneuver that guinea pigs do when they are excited. She would jump several inches off the cushion and, at the apex of the leap, spin around and land facing a different direction. Then she would shrug her shoulders, and a ripple would pass through her small body as if to say, "Wow! This feels so good!" And then she would do it again. This never failed to bring peals of laughter from me, which was another reason why she so reminded me of a jester entertaining at court.

But my laughter soon stopped and turned to alarm as she took a leap upward, spun around, and missed the hassock. With a thud she landed on the hardwood floor and lay there on her belly, legs splayed out, chin on the floor, and eyes open, stunned. I was at her side in an instant, feeling guilty that I had been negligent in my duties as a guinea pig mother, and looked her over without moving her.

All her legs and her head seemed to be in the right places; even her spine was straight I noticed thankfully. But as I looked closer, I could see a spot of blood on the floor in front of her mouth. I crouched low, ear to the floor, and peered intently at her nose, mouth, and chin. One of her incisors, the big front teeth that most animals have, was sticking out between her lips at an odd angle. And on the fur between her bottom lip and chin was a trickle of blood.

I picked her up and cradled her against my chest in the folds of my big sweatshirt on our way to the kitchen sink. Once there, I lay her on a clean towel on the counter and washed my hands. She didn't offer to move as I rinsed the soap off my hands and dried them on another clean towel. I examined her mouth. The incisor was almost entirely dislodged from the socket; it hung from the upper gum by a strand of tissue. There was little blood, so I did not have to apply direct pressure to her mouth or gum. But she still was not moving, and I was worried about shock. I wrapped her more securely in the towel and lay her in her enclosure while I went to call Marc, our vet.

Before leaving, I dissolved four pillules of Aconite in a dropper bottle of distilled water and gave her a dose, four drops on her lower lip. On the ride over, my son Forrest held her in his lap, wrapped in the towel, and gave her more drops on her lip every ten minutes. Half an hour later, by the time we arrived, we had given her four doses of Aconite and she was no longer acting shocked and stunned. Marc met us at the door to his clinic behind his house.

Following an extensive physical exam, where he listened to her heart, timed her pulse, examined her eyes for the telltale dilation that would indicate a concussion, and checked for broken bones, Marc announced that she was in rather good shape for having fallen from such a high place for a

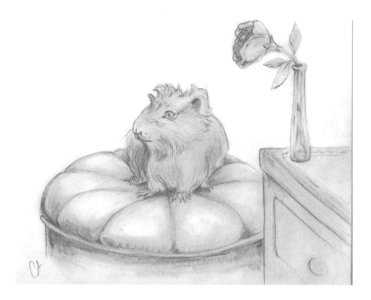

guinea pig. He then turned his attention to her mouth and tooth.

Holding her mouth open with a sterilized paper clip hooked onto her intact upper incisor, he quickly assessed the situation, looking grave and hopeful at the same time. "Two things need attention right away," he began. "First, I'll need to stitch her bottom lip. That's where the small amount of blood is coming from; it looks as though she fell on it and the tooth punctured the soft tissues when she landed.

"Second, because this is an important tooth for an animal of her species, I want to try to save it. The tooth's not fractured as far as I can tell, and that's really in her favor. It looks like it's simply dislodged from the socket. The root is still there, I can see it sticking up out of the top of the tooth. That's also a good thing, because if I implant it back into the gum, it's likely that it will reattach to the soft tissue of the gum and probably quickly, too."

"How are you going to secure the tooth in place while it is healing?" I asked. "And how will she eat during the time that the tooth is growing back into place?" I also wanted to know.

"There's a simple technique we can utilize to save her tooth. I want to splint it into place with wire and dental acrylic, attaching it to the adjacent tooth. It will make a strong bond, and hold it secure while the root is reestablishing itself."

"Dental acrylic? What's that?"

"It's a form of plastic compound that can be painted on and around teeth. It will harden in a few minutes after application, creating a very hard bond. Almost like superglue," Marc added with a smile. "I'll use very small gauge wire to splint the tooth next to its twin, then cover both teeth and the wire with the acrylic bonding material."

I was concerned that the bonding material with the wire imbedded in it would become a permanent fixture in her mouth, and said so. "It might be possible for it to become permanent," Marc began to explain. "Dental acrylic is used in human dentistry all the time to permanently fill in chips in teeth that are injured as the result of various accidents. But an interesting characteristic of this compound is that the longer it remains on a dental surface, the harder it becomes and the more firm the bond. Amnesia's tooth will, I hope, be firmly rooted before the acrylic hardens into a permanent material. When the root is firmly embedded and the surrounding gum tissue has contracted around the base of the tooth, and the time comes to remove the splint and the acrylic, I'll grind it off with a special dental grinding tool I have."

"But what about feeding her?" I asked again. "Won't she have a hard time eating her favorite burdock root and carrots?"

"You'll have to give her grain mashes and very tiny grated pieces of roots for a while. Just chop them up. The incisors are used by those animals that have them to flake and chew off smaller pieces of roots that can be easily ground up by the back molars. You'll have extra kitchen duty, that's sure. But that's small penance for your error, and you should be really happy that we have the option of saving her tooth and that she's not more seriously injured."

The lecture that I had been dreading followed. "You know better than to let her play on surfaces that are so high off the floor. Everything else you do with her is fine. Goodness, she has a great life for a little animal; you dote on her like she was one of your own. But in this one thing you have done her no favor. Wherever she was is a place that's now and forever off limits." Appropriately chastised, I nodded in mute agreement and stroked Amnesia's ears in silent apology.

I passed the next two hours in the waiting room. When Marc strode through the surgery doors, carrying Amnesia in the towel, he was smiling. "She came through the surgery very well. It was just as I thought; the tooth reimplanted very easily and is now secure with wire and dental acrylic. It will be a couple of hours before the anesthetic wears off, but you can take her home in the meantime. I want you to call me in the morning and let me know how she's doing.

"I will want to know if she's still groggy from the anesthetic and if the swelling in her bottom lip has reduced. You're also going to have to replace her water bottle with a heavy dish; she won't be able to sip comfortably from the metal spout, and I don't want her bumping that tooth. I'll also want to know if she's drinking from the new dish." Marc put a warm, comforting hand on my shoulder. "Okay?"

I nodded and reached out to take Amnesia in my arms, thankful that she was going to be all right and resolved to be more careful of her whereabouts. "Call in the morning," Marc said from the steps as I climbed into my car. "And make an appointment with Petra at the desk to bring her back in a week, okay?"

At home, snuggled into the sleeping corner of her hutch, Amnesia slept the night through. I sat in the wicker chair I had brought in from the sunporch, watching her. It was humbling and painful to admit to myself that my carelessness had caused her accident. Yet there it was; it was my fault, and now it was up to me to see that she recovered and that she had safer places to play.

The next morning, after hand-feeding her shredded burdock root and a wet mash of guinea pig pellets, I called Marc to report on Amnesia's progress. She was doing well. The swelling of her lower lip was almost entirely gone. She seemed quite alert and ate and drank from her dish with her usual gusto. She did have a bit of trouble with closing her lips together, as the wire and dental acrylic made a slight bulge that she was unused to, but Marc was pleased with her progress and indicated that she would soon become accustomed to the new bulge of her front teeth. In response to my question, Marc thought that it would be all right to put a dose of Arnica in her water bowl, to resolve any lingering tenderness. He then reminded me to make an appointment with Petra for a follow-up.

The week before our return visit passed quickly. Amnesia was confined mostly to her hutch, except on evenings when she would sit in my lap on the floor while I watched the evening news. Afterward, we would play together on the kitchen floor, rolling Ping-Pong balls back and forth and attending to her evening grooming sessions. These she particularly enjoyed, rolling over on her back so I could comb the hair on her chest and stomach.

Stretched out like this, I could easily see that the small cut in her lower lip was healing rapidly. I could also see her reimplanted tooth as gravity pulled her upper lip down and back and her mouth hung open.

Two tiny strands of wire held it securely to its twin, the ends of which had been bent over and covered in the bonding compound. I was glad that Marc had thought of this; I had been concerned that the ends of the wire would abrade the soft tissue lining the inside of her upper lip. The dental bonding material was only painted into the cleft between the teeth, gluing them together. It was a masterly job. I was glad to have such a skilled and competent vet for my animal companions.

Thursday came—the day of our appointment. Marc used the sterilized paper clip again to hold Amnesia's mouth open. This time she was anesthetized and lay on her side on the exam table. He had already removed the single stitch in her lower lip and declared that wound totally healed.

"This is great," Marc said, gently pushing on the tooth with a gloved finger. "The tooth is firmly implanted and the wire and excess bonding compound can be removed." "Excess? What do you mean excess?" I asked, a nervous edge tinging my voice.

"It's okay," Marc reassured me with confidence. "I'll remove the wire along with most of the bonding acrylic, but leave the material intact where the two teeth are now joined together. It will make them stronger than they were originally, and also impervious to decay or chipping where the acrylic covers the enamel."

Over the grinding noise of the dental tool, Marc inquired about our new television viewing arrangements.

"I gave the hassock to the Lady's Auxiliary Club for their summer yard sale. I have to admit that I was quite attached to it. It was my great-grandmother's you know. I used to sit on it at her feet while she tatted; nobody does that anymore. It's almost a lost art now."

Marc's eyebrows wrinkled in perplexity. "Like miniature macrame," I explained, enjoying the reversal of our roles for a brief moment. "Doilies and such. From France, I think. European anyway. At any rate, it was too much of a temptation to have the stool in the house, and I felt that having it around would confuse Amnesia about why she wasn't allowed to get up on it anymore. We sit on the floor on pillows. And surrounded by them, too."

"All done," Marc said, stepping back and surveying his work. Amnesia's two upper incisors gleamed whitely, side by side and straight as they ever were. One small paw stuck up in the air, bent limply at the wrist. She looked much as she always did when she fell asleep on her back in the corner of her hutch.

"I remember my great-grandmother, too," Marc said, placing Amnesia in my arms. "She had this saying she always quoted whenever she dropped anything."

I waited for the punch line that always announced the end of our visits.

"It can't fall any further than the floor," Marc quipped through a big smile.

FIRST AID FOR TEETH INJURIES

IF A TOOTH IS DISLODGED FROM THE SOCKET
If bleeding is severe, *apply direct pressure.*
>   Firmly press a clean, dry pad or cloth to the wound (if you have no pad, use your hand).
> Keep pressing firmly, enough to make bleeding stop. If pad becomes soaked, put a second pad on top of the first and press harder. *Do not* remove first pad—this interrupts clotting action.
> Keep pressing until bleeding stops or help is obtained.
> Raise bleeding part higher than the heart to slow bleeding.
> Treat for shock (cover the animal to retain body heat).
> Place the tooth in a clean, airtight plastic bag, along with some saliva from the animal's mouth, and take it with the animal to your veterinarian. Your vet may be able to reimplant it.

Seek veterinary attention immediately.

HOMEOPATHY FOR TEETH INJURIES

Status always critical: *Seek veterinary attention immediately.* Give doses of four pellets at five- to ten-minute intervals en route to your veterinarian.

Symptoms	Remedy
Sudden acute trauma, may be bleeding, shock or fear	Aconite (consider Nature's Rescue*)
Always consider for pain and bruising	Arnica
Copious bleeding; watery, bright red blood	Phos

*Dilute four drops in an ounce of water and give four drops of this mixture on tongue or lips. Or hold open bottle under the nose, as with smelling salts. May be repeated as needed until calm is restored.

CHAPTER 37
Vomiting

Anyone who has ever lived with an animal has encountered this troubling complaint. As unpleasant as it is for us as caregivers to clean up the aftermath, rest assured that it is even more unpleasant for the animal who has suffered it. My best advice for dealing with vomiting is threefold: use lots of paper toweling and air freshener, if necessary; be kind and understanding (it wasn't done intentionally to annoy you); and if the trouble persists, consult your veterinarian to find out the underlying cause.

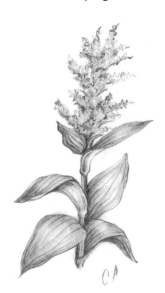

Hellabore plant

FIRST AID FOR VOMITING

CAUSES OF VOMITING

Acute gastritis (acute inflammation of the stomach lining)

Symptoms

Lack of appetite

Lethargy

Vomiting of food or water or both

Fever is usually absent; if fever accompanies vomiting, this may be a serious disease. Consult your veterinarian.

CAUSES

Dietary upsets, menu changes

Choose a remedy from the list.

Foreign object swallowed

Seek veterinary attention immediately.

Food allergy or sensitivity

Choose a remedy from the list.

Feed a bland diet until symptoms subside.

Overeating (puppies)

Feed smaller portions.

Parasites

Consult your veterinarian.

Poisoning

Seek veterinary attention immediately.

Acute gastric syndrome, also known as gastric bloat (overdistention of the stomach accompanied by too much acidity and spasms of the cardiac and pyloric sphincters). *Seek veterinary attention immediately.*

Symptoms (rapidly escalate after a few hours of onset and become life-threatening), in order of appearance.

Unproductive retching or very little mucus raised

Extremely swollen abdomen

Difficulty breathing

Pale mucous membranes of the eyes, mouth

Restlessness and discomfort

Drooling, prostration

Note: These symptoms can lead to death. *Seek veterinary attention immediately.*

Causes

Excessive consumption of food or water; in grass-eaters, impacted fodder or hay

Swallowing of large quantities of air

Barbiturate anesthesia

Stress

Treatment

Surgical intervention

Gastric torsion (twisted stomach or bowel)—see Chapter 13 on colic and *seek veterinary attention immediately.*

Symptoms

Almost the same as acute gastric syndrome, but slower in development

May be seen in ruminants and deep-chested dogs, such as Irish setters and Great Danes

Causes

Produced by a 180-degree twist of the stomach

Treatment

Surgical intervention

FIRST AID FOR SIMPLE STOMACH UPSET

Rest the stomach

Non-grass-eaters only: Fast the animal for twenty-four hours.

Grass-eaters only: Feed small amount of chopped hay. Many animals such as ruminants cannot vomit (like cows, horses, rabbits, and guinea pigs).

All food goes in one direction only: out through the intestinal tract. If horses, cows, goats, or sheep display stomach or digestive difficulties and stop eating, *seek veterinary attention immediately.*

All animals: Provide adequate fluid intake.

Give and follow instructions for electrolyte solution in the recipe section.

All animals: Choose a homeopathic remedy from the list and follow instructions for dosage frequency.

HOMEOPATHY FOR VOMITING

Status critical: *Seek veterinary attention immediately.* Give doses of four pellets at five- to ten-minute intervals en route to your veterinarian.

Status acute: After an initial dose (four pellets), dosing may be repeated at half-hourly intervals for up to four doses or until condition is relieved. If there is no response, consult your veterinarian.

Status chronic: After an initial dose (four pellets), continue with two doses a day or until symptoms subside. If there is no response, consult your veterinarian.

SYMPTOMS	REMEDY
Vomiting and diarrhea from spoiled food; animal is cold, chilly, sweaty, agitated; great thirst, takes frequent, small sips of cold water.	Ars (follow with electrolyte solution*)
Vomiting of green fluid; useful in colic or teething; animal is cramped, doubles up with pain diarrhea green, hot, foul, slimy.	Cham (follow with electrolyte solution)
Vomiting, abdomen very painful to touch; slimy salivation; hiccups and intense thirst for cold drinks	Merc (follow with electrolyte solution)
Hysterical vomiting from emotional upset or fright	Nat mur (follow with electrolyte solution)
Vomiting from rich food; mouth dry, thirstless; drowsy	Nux vom (follow with electrolyte solution)
Undigested food vomited just after swallowing; water vomited after warming in stomach; postoperative	Phos

vomiting; stomach painful to the touch;
symptoms worse from touch or physical
exertion; symptoms better with cold,
open air, sleep

*See Appendix for recipe.

Appendix

KITTEN AND PUPPY
MILK REPLACEMENT FORMULA

8 oz. evaporated milk
8 oz. fresh water
one egg yolk (do not use egg white)
1 tbsp. corn syrup (prevents diarrhea)

Blend together. Store refrigerated in a clean glass jar. Warm only amount to be used (just warm to the touch).

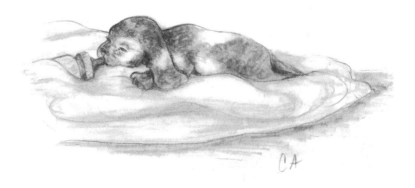

SPECIAL NOTES ON FEEDING ORPHANED YOUNG

FEEDING FREQUENCY (AS A GENERAL RULE INFANT CARNIVORES ARE FED EVERY TWO TO THREE HOURS FOR AT LEAST SIXTEEN HOURS A DAY)

Birth to two weeks old: formula every two hours
Three weeks old: formula every three hours and introduction of semisolids into formula by addition of baby cereals, cat food, and other foods, making a thin gruel
Four to five weeks old: formula every four hours
Five weeks old and older: formula three times a day
Wean to all-solid diet at about six weeks old.

FEEDING AMOUNT

As a general rule, feed only as much as fills the belly, so that the abdomen is slightly plump, not distended. The tummy will feel slightly rounded when lightly rubbed.
Newborn, four to eight ounces body weight: two to four tablespoons of formula per feeding
Ten to twenty-four ounces body weight: four to eight ounces of formula per feeding

FEEDING POSITION

Do not feed a carnivore infant on its back. The proper position for feeding with a bottle or dropper is resting on its stomach with head elevated. Some kittens and puppies get air in their stomachs when nursing, and burping (as with human infants) is helpful. It is also helpful to gently massage the infant's stomach during and after feeding.

ELECTROLYTE SOLUTION RECIPE

1 quart clean water (no chlorine or flouride)
1 tbsp. sugar or honey
1 tsp. common table salt

Mix well and refrigerate unused portions in a clean container. Warm only amount to be used to room temperature before use. Electrolyte solution that is left out will turn mouldy. For extended use, make a fresh batch every day.

Electrolyte solution replenishes lost body fluids. Severely dehydrated animals may have lost fluids equivalent to 10 percent of their body weight. Less acute dehydration may be helped by simply offering as much electrolyte solution as the animal will drink on its own, either in a bowl or from an eyedropper. The following standard amounts should be given over the course of a day until the animal is drinking on its own from its water bowl.

DAILY STANDARD INTAKES FOR ELECTROLYTE SOLUTION

Kittens and puppies: three tablespoons
Animals weighing five pounds: four to five tablespoons
Animals weighing ten pounds: three quarters of a cup
Animals weighing fifteen or more pounds: one quarter of a
cup for each five pounds body weight.

SPECIAL NOTES ON BIRDS, REPTILES, AND FISH

BIRDS

All remedies and first-aid suggestions in this manual are applicable to all species. With birds, administration of any first-aid treatment should be conducted with standard bird-handling techniques in mind.

Do not administer fluids by mouth (beak), since birds are prone to aspiration (inhalation) of fluids, which may lead to serious respiratory problems. Instead, one drop of any remedy dose, diluted in distilled water, or Nature's Rescue diluted in distilled water, may be placed directly in the eye. For birds, the standard dose is one single drop. A repeat dose is also a single drop (in the eye).

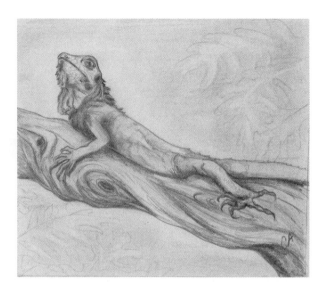

REPTILES

All remedies and first-aid suggestions in this manual are applicable to all species. With regard to reptiles and amphibians, administration of any first-aid treatment should be conducted with standard reptile-handling techniques in mind.

It may be difficult to administer pillules or liquids to reptiles via the mouth, since they are prone to biting or are delicate enough to warrant very gentle handling. As with birds, a drop may be easily administered to the eye. Reptiles, and especially amphibians, also absorb moisture through the skin, and a diluted remedy or dilution of Nature's Rescue rubbed or dropped on the skin will be directly absorbed.

FISH

As with other species, homeopathic remedies are helpful with problems affecting fish. To use them, simply place a standard dose in the tank water. But dilute the remedy in a measuring cup full of water taken from the tank before adding it to the tank water, so as to keep the environmental temperature constant. Slow growth, fear, fright and panic, loss of appetite, and skin (scale) and fin problems (including parasites) will be most commonly encountered. While homeopathic remedies can be helpful with health problems encountered in fish, their delicate physical structure and physiology require diagnosis and treatment by a veterinarian specializing in diseases and health issues affecting fish.

SUGGESTED FIRST-AID EQUIPMENT

A cardboard carton for emergency transport or an animal transport
    case with a removable top
Clean towels
Hydrogen peroxide
Distilled water
Tincture of iodine or merthiolate
Arnica oil or gel
Bag Balm
Sterile gauze pads, cotton balls, and cotton swabs
A plastic eyedropper
Small, blunt-nosed scissors
Elastic bandages for sprains
White waterproof adhesive tape
Plastic temperature strip (for taking the temperature)
Calendula tincture or ointment
A preassembled kit of the remedies used in this text, available from
    Homeopathy Overnight (see Resources)

Bibliography

Biddis, K. J. *Homeopathy in Veterinary Practice.* Essex, England: C. W. Daniel Co., 1987.

Boericke, William. *Materia Medica with Repertory,* 9th ed. Philadelphia: Boericke and Tafel, 1927.

Boger, C. M. *A Synoptic Key to the Materia Medica.* New Delhi: B. Jain Publishers, 1993.

Chapman, J. B., and Edward L. Perry. *Biochemic Theory and Practice,* rev. ed. St. Louis: Formur Incorporated Publishers, 1976.

Day, Christopher. *The Homeopathic Treatment of Small Animals: Principles and Practice.* New Delhi: B. Jain Publishers, 1988.

Farrington, Harvey. *Homeopathy and Homeopathic Prescribing.* New Delhi: B. Jain Publishers, 1993.

Fowler, Murray A., ed. *Zoo and Wild Animal Medicine.* Philadelphia: W. B. Saunders Company, 1986.

Fraser, C. M., ed. *The Merck Veterinary Manual,* 6th ed. Rathway, N. J.: Merck & Co., 1986.

Gibson, Douglas. *Studies of Homeopathic Remedies.* Bucks, England: Beaconsfield Publishers, 1987.

Macleod, George. *A Veterinary Materia Medica and Clinical Repertory with a Materia Medica of the Nosodes.* Great Britain: C. W. Daniel Co., 1989.

————. *Cats: Homeopathic Remedies.* Essex, England: C. W. Daniel Co., 1990.

Moore, James. *Dog Diseases.* New Delhi: B. Jain Publishers, 1991.

Ruddock, Edward H. *The Pocket Manual of Homeopathy; Veterinary Medicine.* New Delhi: B. Jain Publishers, 1989.

Rush, John. *The Hand-Book to Veterinary Homeopathy or the Homeopathic Treatment of the Horse, the Ox, the Sheep, the Dog and the Swine.* New Delhi: B. Jain Publishers, 1990.

Wildlife Rescue, Inc. *Outline for Mammal Care* (employee handout). Palo Alto, Calif.: Wildlife Rescue, Inc., 1985.

Wolff, H. G. *Your Healthy Cat: Homeopathic Medicines for Common Feline Ailments.* Berkeley, Calif.: North Atlantic Books and Homeopathic Educational Services, 1991.

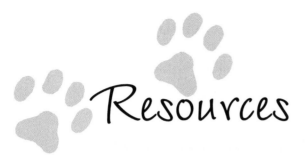

Resources

Boiron/Borneman
6 Campus Boulevard
Building A
Newtown Square, PA 19073
(610) 325-7464 or 800-BOIRON-1
West Coast Branch:
98C West Cochran Street
Simi Valley, CA 93065
(805) 582-9091 or 800-BOIRON-1

Manufacturer of homeopathic remedies.

Homeopathic Educational Services
2124 Kittredge Street
Berkeley, CA 94704
(510) 649-0294 or 800-359-9051 (orders only)

Extensive list of books on homeopathy and related health issues; remedy kits. Free catalog.

Homeopathy Online: A Journal of Homeopathic Medicine
www.lyghtforce.com/HomeopathyOnline

Journal on the worldwide web. (Other homeopathy-related Web

sites exist, but addresses change rapidly. Use a search engine to find the latest sites.)

Homeopathy Overnight
RR1 Box 818
Kingfield, Maine 04947
(800) 276-4223 (ARNICA-3)
Fax: (207) 265-0029

Supplier of preassembled kits specially designed for use with this book, as well as individual remedies. Call for prices and shipping information.

International Foundation for Homeopathy (IFH)
P.O. Box 7
Edmonds, WA 98020
(206) 776-4147
Fax: 206-776-1499

A nonprofit organization dedicated to the education of professional homeopaths according to the highest standards of classical homeopathy. Activities include professional courses, an annual conference, and bimonthly magazine. Referrals to graduates of the (IFH) professional course will be provided with a SASE.

National Center for Homeopathy (NCH)
801 North Fairfax Street
Suite 306
Alexandria, VA 22314
(703)548-7790
Fax: 703-548-7792
nchinfo@igc.apc.org

A nonprofit membership organization dedicated to promoting homeopathy in the U.S. through education, publication, research, and membership sevices. Membership is $40/year and includes the monthly magazine *Homeopathy Today* and the annual directory of practitioners, study groups, and resources. The directory lists licensed health-care professionals who devote 25 to 100 percent of their practice to homeopathy. An information packet, which includes the directory, is available to nonmembers for $6. The directory is also available at http://www.healthy.net/nch.

Standard Homeopathic Company
154 West 131 Street
Box 61067
Los Angeles, CA 90061
(800) 624-9659 or (213) 321-4284

Manufacturer of a full line of homeopathic medicines in various dosage forms, including tincture, dilution, pellets, and tablets.

Index

OTHER BOOKS ON HOMEOPATHY
FROM HEALING ARTS PRESS

The Family Homeopath: Safe, Natural, and Effective Health Care for You and Your Children
Robin Hayfield
ISBN 0-89281-532-9

Handbook of Homeopathy
Gerhard Koehler
ISBN 0-89281-345-8

Homeopathic Medicine: A Doctor's Guide to Remedies for Common Ailments
Trevor Smith, M.D.
ISBN 0-89281-293-1

Homeopathic Medicine: First Aid and Emergency Care
Lyle W. Morgan, Ph.D.
ISBN 0-89281-249-4

Homeopathic Medicine for Mental Health
Trevor Smith, M.D.
ISBN 0-89281-291-5

Homeopathic Medicine for Women: An Alternative Approach to Gynecological Health Care
Trevor Smith, M.D.
ISBN 0-89281-236-2

Homeopathic Treatment of Sports Injuries
Lyle W. Morgan, Ph.D.
ISBN 0-89281-227-3

Homeopathy: From Alchemy to Medicine
Elizabeth Danciger
ISBN 0-89281-290-7

Homeopathy and Your Child: A Parent's Guide to Homeopathic Treatment from Infancy through Adolescence
Lyle W. Morgan, Ph.D.
ISBN 0-89281-330-X

Homeopathy for Menopause
Beth MacEoin
ISBN 0-89281-648-1

Healing Arts Press is a division of Inner Traditions International.
These books may be ordered by calling 1-800-246-8648.